THE
WILD DIET

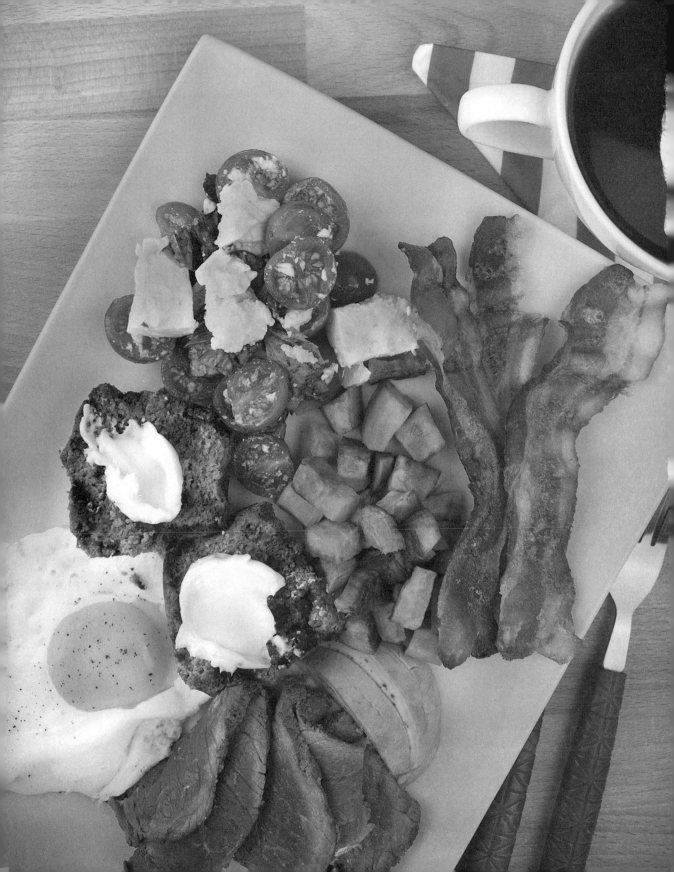

THE
WILD DIET

Go Beyond Paleo to Burn Fat, Beat Cravings,
and Drop 20 Pounds in 40 Days

ABEL JAMES

AVERY · AN IMPRINT OF PENGUIN RANDOM HOUSE · NEW YORK

an imprint of Penguin Random House LLC
375 Hudson Street
New York, New York 10014

Most Avery books are available at special quantity discounts for bulk purchase for sales promotions, premiums, fund-raising, and educational needs. Special books or book excerpts also can be created to fit specific needs. For details, write SpecialMarkets@penguinrandomhouse.com.

Photographs © 2015 by Melinda Bryce

Excerpt on pages 347–349: Originally published in the December 1965 *Ladies' Home Journal* ® magazine

The Library of Congress has catalogued the hardcover edition as follows:

James, Abel.
The wild diet : get back to your roots, burn fat, and drop up to 20 pounds in 40 days/Abel James.
p.   cm.
ISBN 978-1-58333-573-4
1. High-protein diet—Recipes.   2. Reducing diets—Recipes.
3. Prehistoric peoples—Nutrition.   4. Cooking (Wild foods).   I. Title
RM237.65.J36   2015   2014047008
641.5'638—dc23

ISBN 978-1-10198-286-0 (paperback)

Printed in the United States of America
7   9   10   8   6

BOOK DESIGN BY MEIGHAN CAVANAUGH

DEDICATION AND A TOAST

This book is dedicated to my grandparents
Marion and Horace Bascom

From Our Family to Yours: Nan's Favorite Toast

"HERE'S TO THEE AND THY FOLKS

FROM ME AND MY FOLKS.

SURE THERE NEVER WAS FOLKS

SINCE FOLKS WAS FOLKS,

EVER LOVED ANY FOLKS

HALF AS MUCH AS ME AND MY FOLKS

LOVE THEE AND THY FOLKS!"

Wild |wīld| *adjective (of an animal or plant)*
Living or growing in the natural environment; not domesticated or
cultivated. Passionate, vehement, unrestrained. Untamed.

"Wild with excitement."

Di·et |dī-it| *noun*
The kinds of food that a person, animal, or community habitually eats.

"The native human diet."

AUTHOR'S NOTE

Earlier this year, my wife, Alyson, and I dined at a farm-to-table restaurant in Florida with twenty leaders in the health movement, a motley crew of bestselling authors, nutritionists, Olympians, cooks, and physicians. After a long week, we were ready for a feast.

Our waiter scribbled furiously as Alyson, my cute-as-a-button, 105-pound wife, and I ordered:

- Bacon deviled eggs
- Two roasted marrow bones with local herbs and spices
- Two hearty farm-fresh salads with aged meat, nuts, and avocado
- Charcuterie board with a trio of duck, lamb, and pork pâtés; raw artisanal cheese; and a side of homemade sauerkraut
- Sautéed sweetbreads
- Wild sea bass with mushroom butter sauce
- Grass-fed sirloin steak (medium-rare, of course) with heirloom vegetables

As others watched in awe, we polished off the lot, including more than our fair share of wine and champagne. One of the health experts said with a gasp, "How on earth do you two eat so much and stay so lean?"

This book is the answer to that question.

I hope you enjoy it.

In health and happiness,
Abel James Bascom

CONTENTS

INTRODUCTION:
BAND GONE WILD

As we hop aboard Tim McGraw's tour bus idling outside a Quality Inn in Austin, Texas, I suddenly realize that being healthy is cool again.

Instead of smoking ashtrays, passed-out groupies, and stale beer, the smell of strong coffee wafts through the country superstar's Zen-like tour bus. A veritable cornucopia of fresh produce, organic seaweed snacks, and an imposing 5-pound sack of Brazil nuts fill the mini-kitchen. Despite filming the *Today* show in New York City twenty-four hours earlier, these road warriors are bright-eyed and bushy-tailed. Denny, enjoying an unprecedented twenty-year reign as Tim's guitarist and musical director, introduces us to the rest of the band.

Fresh off his feature on the cover of *Men's Health* after losing 40 pounds, forty-seven-year-old Tim McGraw is a specimen of health. He credits his pumped-up biceps and six-pack abs to his band's new routine of clean eating and intense outdoor workouts on the road. His tour bus even pulls a trailer dedicated to unconventional exercise gear—hauling heavy chains, sledgehammers, and sandbags across the country.

"Whoa, the Fat-Burning Man. . . . It's so surreal you're here!" Deano, the fiddle player, muses, somehow expressing precisely how I feel at that moment. I'm not sure exactly when it happened, but more people seem to know me as "Fat-Burning Man," the tongue-in-cheek title of my hit health show, than as the road-weary musician I've been for most of my life. I'd taken time away from music to focus on inspiring others to live better by eating real food and breaking a good sweat. As far as I was concerned, I was just a regular guy babbling into a microphone on my computer and doing my best to make my show valuable to whoever happened to be tuning in. It wasn't until I received my favorite thank-you note ever from a musician named Denny that I realized people were actually *listening*. Better yet, these newfound health nuts were actually getting results that blew my mind.

A loyal listener of *Fat-Burning Man*, Denny has been following the Wild Diet for more than a year. Enjoying hearty meals that include plenty of butter, bacon, and eggs, he's dropped 46 pounds. Impressed by Denny's transformation, several bandmates came along for the ride.

"Billy, our keyboard player, only decided to try the Wild Diet because he's allowed to eat coffee cake." Denny grins. "It really isn't that complicated—you just listen to your body and eat when you're hungry. It's great. I'm full of energy and feel fifteen years younger."

"My kids love eating this way," adds Deano. "They're totally into organ meats and headcheese. Their friends think eating brains is cool."

After Deano convinces us to taste his latest culinary fascination, emu oil (it's not bad, actually), we take Denny back to our place to play a few tunes. On the way, we grab two cups of fresh-roasted "fatty coffee" (see page 249) with butterfat and pure cocoa, our first "meal" of the day. To fuel an epic jam session, we polish off a few pints of green smoothie, sample asparagus and bacon quiche, and indulge in homemade blueberry muffins, pumpkin scones, and Alyson's newest cheesecake recipe (Peanut Butter Chocolate "Cheesecake" with Hazelnut Crust—try it yourself on page 250) with our afternoon tea. A few hours later, our luxurious dinner includes bacon-wrapped sea scallops, wild Atlantic salmon, creamed spinach with toasted prosciutto, and a wee bit of wine. This ain't no ordinary diet.

Sound incredible? Well, the truth is that I haven't always had the body of an underwear model while feasting like a rock star. Before people knew me as my fat-burning alter ego whose abs are plastered all over the Internet, I was the chubby kid with chipmunk cheeks.

I've always loved food. As a toddler in the eighties, I discovered that the spiral cord on our kitchen phone didn't quite reach the candy cupboard. So every time the phone rang, I sprinted to the candy and drooled like Pavlov's dog. As soon as Mom picked up the phone, now safely out of reach, I'd stuff my face with as much chocolate, candy, and cookies as humanly possible.

One night, still dressed in my suspenders and bow tie after playing clarinet at the local diner for pocket money, my dad took me aside for an important talk.

"Abel, your body is about to go through some changes," he explained with a gentle smile. "With our genes, you can grow up to be overweight . . . or strong and athletic. It all depends on how you eat and exercise in the next few years as you grow into a teenager."

An athletic strapping stonemason for most of his life, Dad had packed on nearly 30 pounds after he was forced into a desk job when the economy tanked. I listened closely and took heed. I didn't want to be overweight, and for the first time in my life I realized I had a choice. And then I was off.

I learned in one of Dad's magazines that "fat makes you fat and clogs your arteries." So I declared that I would switch to fat-free milk, shun red meat, and I even started to carry around extra napkins to sponge the grease off pizza in order to avoid excess cholesterol. I was eight years old.

I took up every sport I could. A little too excited after watching *Rocky* for the first time, I choked down a full glass of raw eggs before my morning workout and chased chickens around the backyard. I cranked the brittle gears of my yard-sale Huffy to the summit of the legendary Piper Hill and trained like a Ninja Turtle to get my purple belt in karate. By seventh grade, my baby fat and chipmunk cheeks grew into a chiseled frame with a strong jaw to match. The girls even started calling me "Mr. Buff," my first stupid nickname.

I'd done it—the chubby kid who played clarinet at Christmas parties had transformed into a handsome, athletic teen. But getting fat doesn't happen all at once. Sometimes it sneaks up on you.

After speeding through Dartmouth College, studying brain science, music, and technology, it was time to pay off a few nasty student loans and chase the American Dream. Turning down offers from Wall Street and the CIA, I took a job as a strategy consultant for Fortune 500s in Washington, D.C., moonlighting as a computer programmer. I quickly learned that spending nearly all of my waking hours under fluorescent lights takes its toll. But there was work to be done, loans to be paid, and no time for hikes in the woods.

My fancy new office had a "Healthy Snacks" program to help us get through the long hours consulting with the bigwigs. I was pleased to find that many of the snacks lined up perfectly with the fat-free, low-calorie diet praised by the media and health magazines. I nibbled on fat-free whole-grain crackers, nonfat yogurt, and zero-calorie Jell-O, and I sipped cholesterol-free soy milk; cloudy, experimental diet soda; and other oddities provided by our Fortune 500 clients in the food and beverage industry.

When I sat down with my new physician for my first checkup as an adult, he avoided eye contact at first, shuffling papers on his desk. His brow suddenly furrowed as he looked up at me with a wide-eyed grin.

"You have *great* insurance!" he blurted.

From that point on, I peed in a cup and had my blood drawn every time I set foot in the doctor's office, which was often. My results didn't look good. I had high blood pressure, high cholesterol, elevated triglycerides, thyroid problems, insomnia, and many other disorders and diseases of civilization that we're somehow conditioned to "expect" as our youth evades us.

"You have the body of a middle-aged man," the doctor admitted grimly. "With your blood pressure and family history, you might be looking at heart disease, thyroid disorder, and even diabetes if you don't cut out dietary fat and do more cardio starting right now."

Doc put me on a new painkiller for a running injury, a prescription-strength antiperspirant, several sleep meds, and even an antidepressant that he promised would "help me sleep."

Gritting my teeth, I followed the doc's advice. I popped the pills, counted every last calorie, grew accustomed to constant hunger, nibbled on low-fat food that tasted like cardboard, and jogged five times a week.

I proudly became a vegetarian, swapped real butter for zero-cholesterol vegetable oil spread, and replaced farm-fresh eggs with 100% whole wheat bagels with nonfat cream cheese and zero-calorie jam from the supermarket. Without fresh veggies from our family's garden, I stocked up on bananas, 100% orange juice (with pulp, obviously), and reduced-sodium canned vegetable juice from the Safeway down the street.

But every time I went to see my doctor, I was fatter and sicker than ever . . . and people started to notice. Subtlety was never my boss's strong suit. One day, he just laid it right out there.

"Whoa, Abel, you've put on a few pounds! What *happened* to you? Too many sweets, eh?" Nope—I was dieting harder than ever.

I took a good, hard look in the mirror and I didn't like what I saw.

Instead of a strong, vital twenty-four-year-old, I had the flab of an unhealthy man twice my age. The impossibly low-fat diet recommended by doctors, diet books, magazines, and the media didn't appear to be working. Fed up, I diverted my energy to healing myself. I scoured medical textbooks, underground bodybuilding manuals, and the nooks and crannies of the Internet to find the perfect protocol to drop my excess fat and regain my vitality.

I quickly discovered that everything I thought I knew about diet was wrong.

When I started my new "diet," I did the opposite of what most well-meaning nutritionists might tell you. I chowed down on the most delicious and rich foods of my life— real butter, scrambled eggs, fresh veggies, rich meats, coconut, aged cheese, steak, and chocolate. I flushed my pharmaceuticals and called my mom, an author and herbalist, once a week to reincorporate adaptogenic herbs, teas, and tonics back into my daily habits.

HERE'S WHAT HAPPENED . . .

The mounting health problems that I'd been told were just part of getting older—high blood pressure, heartburn, low energy, thyroid issues, insomnia, dry skin, acne, kidney stones, the spare tire, and much more—quickly improved. My sugar cravings, nagging hunger, and mood swings gently faded with each passing week. I began to feel a glowing energy and clarity that reminded me of what it was like to be a young buck in his prime. My double chin quickly receded, and my belly fat followed close behind.

When I stepped on the scale, I was shocked. I had lost 20 pounds of flab in forty days. This fat loss revealed a muscular body and washboard abs that could be slapped right on the cover of a fitness magazine. More important, I had more energy and gusto than I'd felt in my entire life.

But as much as I enjoyed taking my new abs for a spin, I was angry. Why had I been trying so hard to stay on an expensive diet that was making me fat and sick for all those years? Everybody deserves to feel this way.

So I wrote a fat-loss manual and printed twenty copies at Kinko's to send to friends and family. After ten weeks, my dad, cousins, friends, coworkers, and bandmates each dropped around 20 pounds. Even my dental hygienist eventually lost more than 60 pounds by going Wild, just through what I could mumble during my cleanings every six months.

REAL FOOD, REAL RESULTS

After transforming my own body, I launched my health show, *Fat-Burning Man,* to educate and inspire others to be happy and healthy by optimizing their bodies with real food, and cutting-edge science and technology. I had a goal to change a million lives with real food and Wild movement, and word quickly spread. Within the first year, we hit that goal, and even beat out Jillian Michaels, head trainer on *The Biggest Loser*, for Apple's number-one-rated podcast in health. Eventually, the series hit number one in more than eight countries around the world and won four awards in independent media, including Best Health and Fitness Podcast at the Podcast Awards.

If you like this book, you'll enjoy the *Fat-Burning Man* show. I cover almost every subject in this book—from digestion to dead lifts—with detailed, topical interviews with top experts. You can listen in and watch the entire series for free at FatBurningMan.com.

In *The Wild Diet*, you'll find that we are not meant to starve ourselves or count calories. We're wired to eat and live well without getting fat. That's what we've been doing effortlessly for thousands of years, in fact, before we started following the wrong advice.

If you think that you're stuck with the genes you inherited and there's nothing you can do about it, read closely. *The Wild Diet* paints a different picture, one in which we have the power to influence our genetic expression by taking control of the environment around us. As a testament to the healing power of fresh food and a good sweat, I've seen my family, friends, fans, and clients lose many hundreds of pounds, reverse degenerative disease, recover from cancer, extend their life-spans, and win Olympic gold medals using the principles you're about to learn.

I made a conscious choice to write this book in layman's terms with minimal cryptic scientific jargon. Rest assured—*The Wild Diet* is based on proven scientific principles and a growing body of peer-reviewed and independent research. But instead of hurling studies and their equal-and-opposite counterparts back and forth, this book gets straight to the point and shows you what works so you can look and feel better than you ever thought possible. If you'd like to do your own homework, please explore the notes section.

Fair warning: Much of what you read in this book may be "controversial" and stand in direct opposition to current conventional wisdom and popular beliefs. While the principles in this program may seem radical today, I believe that they will be the "breakthroughs" of the future. I am confident that if you read this book with an open mind, the knowledge on the following pages will have the power to change your life.

Ready?

Great. Let's get started.

PART I

How "Healthy" Food Made Us Fat and Sick

WHY WE ALL GAINED 30 POUNDS

The average forty-year-old man in 1960 tipped the scale at 166 pounds. Weighing in at 196 pounds, the average man today is 30 pounds heavier.

What happened?

Like many of us, you've probably put on a few pounds over the past few years. And I bet you've tried to do something about it. Maybe you even went on a crash diet, forcing yourself to count every last calorie and buy expensive packaged dinners and a Shake Weight. Fighting through incessant cravings with shocking self-control, you probably even shed a few pounds. But as soon as you stopped depriving yourself, the fat came right back, didn't it? Most diets seem to imply that you can be lean, but only if you're hungry and miserable.

I'm here to tell you that it doesn't have to be like that.

When the Internet gurus tell you to subsist on cabbage soup, eat thirty bananas a day, or pop caffeine pills to melt off belly fat, don't listen. There's a better way to reclaim your youth and vitality. So get ready—I'm going to gently ask you to set aside nearly everything you've been told about diet, nutrition, and health. Many of the strategies and principles of *The Wild Diet* fly in the face of popular beliefs, fad crash diets, and advice from the droning, half-alive "experts" you see on daytime television.

You don't need me to tell you that our collective health seems doomed. Diabetes, cancer, and heart disease, rare until the turn of the twentieth century, are now predicted to affect almost everyone in the developed world at some point in their lifetime. Health care costs are increasingly crippling our economy, and eight-year-old children are weighing in at 300 pounds. One in three U.S. children born in 2000 will become diabetic in their lifetimes; nearly half of minorities are predicted to develop the disease; and the next generation of children is the first in centuries expected to have shorter life-spans than their parents. This is staggering . . . and also completely preventable.

If you're reading this, then conventional wisdom about nutrition and fitness has probably failed you. Confounded by special interests, misinformation from powerful industry lobbyists, and sleazy health and fitness gurus, the lion's share of conventional wisdom about diet and health is wrong, and those who trumpet its claims are misinformed, misguided, or simply misleading you. *The Wild Diet* will teach you to liberate yourself from the gimmickry, half-baked dogma, and empty promises of the diet and fitness industry.

As host of *Fat-Burning Man*, Apple's number-one-rated show, I've interviewed hundreds of the top experts across the world in weight loss, athletic training, physiology, brain science, and even indigenous tribespeople to figure out why America got fat. I quickly realized that losing fat and building muscle isn't a mystery. I've whittled this approach to health down to a few simple, easy-to-follow principles . . . some of which will surely surprise you.

What many seek to accomplish with extreme fad diets and the stapling of stomachs, we will achieve by restoring your mental and physical balance. Instead of fighting against it, we will work *with* your body to improve your health. Despite what you hear from the screaming maws of overcaffeinated weight-loss trainers on reality shows, you'll soon discover that taking pleasure in nourishing your body is essential to your success. You really can be happy and healthy at the same time.

THE SECRET TO FAT LOSS IN ONE SENTENCE

We don't need more diets, more books, or more information. We need trusted, step-by-step strategies from people who know what they're talking about. If you're familiar with my work, you already know that I've never claimed to be an expert or a guru. I'm just a regular guy who has spent the last decade obsessing about nutrition and fitness so you don't have to. And if you're not in the mood to read another diet book front to back, I'll give you the secret to fat loss in one sentence right now:

Stay away from sugar and processed grains, especially in the morning.

Disappointed? Let me give you some good news before you throw this book across the room.

If you've given up some of your favorite foods—like gooey cheese, chocolate, grilled steak, bacon, butter, full-fat cream, eggs, wine, cheesecake, ice cream, or anything else delicious—for the sake of "health," you're about to have a really good time eating this way. If you've exercised for hours a day, gritting your teeth and sweating pure misery, I'm going to teach you how to burn more fat with just minutes of exercise a week. Sound impossible? Take it from the Fat-Burning Man: Burning fat can be a lot of fun.

WHY DIET BOOKS DISAGREE WITH EACH OTHER

When I met with fancypants editors in Manhattan who were interested in publishing *The Wild Diet*, most said something like this: "So, Abel, your program makes a lot of sense. And your fans and followers clearly get great results. But what's *new* about your diet?"

Wrong question.

Take a second and type "diet" into Google. How many results did you get? I'm going to take a wild guess and say 14 bazillion.

Heard of the raw vegan diet? Dieters were arguing about it before we invented the automobile. How about low-carb? Check out "Banting," which became a fat-loss craze in England during the late 1800s. Last year, one of my blog posts went viral after I announced that I'd received a cease-and-desist letter from a fellow Paleo author. He threatened to sue me unless I removed the words "Paleo Diet" from my work because he had trademarked the term to sell supplements. But even the caveman diet has been around since the 1970s—or for the entire duration of human existence, depending on how you look at it.

And if all the fad diets weren't enough, most "scientific discoveries" touted by the media are ridiculous.

SCIENTIFIC DISCOVERY: EGGS ARE GOOD FOR YOU AGAIN!

MAN LOSES 20 POUNDS BY CUTTING OUT HIS STOMACH!

BREAKING NEWS: MUFFIN TOPS ARE ACTUALLY MADE OF MUFFINS!

Here's the truth—there is no such thing as a "new" diet. Anyone who tells you different is trying to sell you something. The philosophy of the Wild Diet is to honor the natural rhythms of your body and get food as close to its source as possible. Know that this is an ancient way of eating, not a new one. This isn't a diet book, but a book about how to reclaim your health by following the laws of nature (with a few delicious recipes to boot).

Some of what you read in this book will seem like no-brainer common sense. Good. We don't need more conflicting information and fads—it's time to get back to fundamentals. Not too long ago, "dieting" and losing weight weren't even considerations, since most people remained lean throughout their lifetimes. Our body isn't an adversary that we must "diet" and "exercise" into submission, but a remarkable biological system that adapts to the way we eat, train, and live.

WHY PROCESSED FOOD IS A WASTE OF YOUR MONEY

Modern food manufacturers have overwhelmed grocery store shelves with foodstuff that is nutrient-poor, rotten, spoiled, dead, old, and tainted with antibiotics, synthetic hormones, and petroleum-based flavors. They saved a buck on cheap ingredients and didn't tell us they ruined our food in the process. Instead of nourishing our bodies with the fresh bounty of small family farms and gardens, we have been conditioned to subsist on marked-up, overhyped industrial-strength Frankenfoods from Fortune 500 corporations.

Since the rise of convenience food following the Second World War, Big Food has cut corners, capitalized on cheap oil, and embraced backward government policy to doctor our food beyond belief. While we continued to eat foods that go by the same names as those made at home by our parents and grandparents, the ingredients quietly shifted: The honey and natural sugars in our sweets, sauces, and sodas became genetically engineered corn syrup; the hand-churned grass-fed butter on our kitchen table became corn oil; wheat was bred into a plant that would be utterly unrecognizable to our ancestors; and the spices that flavored our favorite dishes were pushed out by artificial chemicals from test tubes.

Assembly-line production may work well for the automotive industry, but its ruthless efficiency and profit-based bent don't serve us well when our health is concerned. Factory food may be convenient and "cheap," but it's killing us.

For the titans of industry who run Big Food, the pursuit of short-term profits has trumped good judgment and clouded ethics. After years of tweaking from legions of white-coated technicians and geneticists, the fundamental nature of our food has changed. The land of milk and honey became the land of soy milk and agave nectar. Today, many of the foods we eat "in the pursuit of health" are intentionally designed to encourage overeating.

Have you ever tried a dinky "100-calorie pack" of crackers, cookies, or chips? When you get to the end of the bag (in, if you're like me, about five seconds flat), you want another one, right? But how many times have you eaten a big, juicy apple (usually about 100 calories, by the way) and said to yourself, "Golly, I really want *another apple* right now"? Doesn't happen. Your brain knows when you eat real food. Processed food makes you crave more, so you *buy* more. Real food fills you up.

But the whole point of eating is to get full, isn't it? This is the first time in the history of man that we're tricked into thinking that we want less *food* in our food. We are surrounded by food, but we're nutritionally starving. Nutrient-poor processed foods distort your appetite and cause you to consume more calories than you need. This perpetuates a vicious cycle of stuffing your face but never feeling totally satisfied or nourished.

When you're hungry, your body doesn't necessarily want food; it craves *nutrition*. If you try to quell your hunger with empty calories or doctored food, your brain and body will never really feel totally satisfied. The key is to feed yourself nutrient-dense foods that satiate your hunger. As I'm sure you've noticed, today's concrete jungle of freeze-dried franchises and chain supermarkets can make life a challenge for any aspiring health nut.

In America, our standards for food are shockingly low. This section of the book may surprise or disgust you, but bear with me—you'll see that poor-quality food is easy to avoid once you know what to look for. But first, buckle up—it's about to get bumpy. What I learned as a consultant inside the diet and health industry made my stomach turn.

The Worst Thing Since Sliced Bread

Something happened to our wheat. Although it claims the same name, the hybridized dwarf wheat we eat today does not resemble the whole grain our parents once ate. For thousands of years, we used hardy ancient varieties of wheat like emmer, einkorn, and khorosan to make bread, pasta, and baked foods. However, the mutant, genetically altered grain that makes up 99 percent of the wheat we eat today has been "dwarfed"—it stops growing at just one-third of the height of the massive amber waves of grain our ancestors sang about.

The blunted stems, high yield, and ease of transport of "dwarf" wheat makes it cheap to produce, but it's also less nutritious and difficult to digest. Since agribusiness began genetically altering wheat in 1960, concentrations of zinc, copper, iron, and magnesium in the grain plummeted (19 to 28 percent lower in the years 1968 to 2005, compared to 1845 to 1967). Big Food has bred a wolf into a Chihuahua, but that's just the beginning of the madness.

It's a wonder to comprehend how expansive field grains are manipulated by man and machine into a 100% wheat bagel or hamburger bun. The truth isn't pretty. Let's travel with "dwarf" wheat on its journey from field to sack.

- After machines remove large contaminants like sticks and rocks, wheat endures high-temperature steam conditioning, which prevents the berries from naturally fermenting. Once the chaff is removed, the endosperm, the least nutritious and starchiest part of the wheat, is separated and ground into a fine powder.

- Chlorine, bromates, and azodicarbonamide are chemicals that are banned in Europe but are used widely in America to improve appearance, remove odors, and standardize texture. Bleaching and oxidizing agents (such as benzoyl peroxide, calcium peroxide, nitrogen dioxide, chlorine, or azodicarbonamide) are added to the flour made from the ground endosperm. Since the most nutritious part of the grain has already been removed during processing, the government mandates that food refiners must "enrich" their flour with synthetic vitamins, which can be difficult to absorb.
- The bleached wheat flour sits in containers for one to two months before being packed into sacks or large tanks to be shipped off to consumers or used to make processed food. Since the wheat hasn't been fermented, soaked, or sprouted to remove toxic antinutrients, this flour contains substances that can damage the gut, causing weight gain, autoimmune disorders, and disease.

TINY LITTLE VEGETABLES

We didn't always blast our modern wheat with heat and chemicals. Once upon a time, our grandparents knew well that grains needed to ferment, soak, and sprout before they were nutritious enough to eat.

Sprouting and fermenting grains essentially turns them into tiny, ready-to-eat vegetables that are more easily digested. Sprouting grains increases the amino acid lysine, reduces antinutrients like phytic acid and lectins, disables enzyme inhibitors, and releases enzymes to increase the absorbability of nutrients. Essentially, when you prepare grains (or any other food) the way that nature intended—through fermenting, soaking, sprouting, followed by low-and-slow cooking—you maximize the nutrient density of your food.

So what happens when we turn this modern flour into "heart-healthy, low-fat, whole-grain" bread? Here is a breakdown of store-bought bread with a label that screams in big, flashy typeface, "ALL NATURAL INGREDIENTS" and "NO ARTIFICIAL PRESERVATIVES ADDED":

Enriched bleached wheat flour (bleached wheat flour, malted barley, niacin, reduced iron, thiamine mononitrate, riboflavin), water, high-fructose corn syrup, yeast, wheat bran, vital wheat gluten, butter. Contains 2% or less of each of the following: rye meal, corn flour, molasses, rolled whole wheat, salt, dough conditioners (ammonium sulfate, sodium stearoyl lactylate), brown sugar, honey, vinegar, oatmeal, soy flour, mono- and diglycerides, partially hydrogenated soybean oil.

Here's what you should know about these ingredients:

- Enriched bleached wheat flour is refined white flour. "Enriched" is a confusing term—it sounds healthy, but it's not. The bran and the germ portion of the whole wheat have been refined out, leaving you with the least nutritious and most fattening portion of the wheat. To compensate for refining out approximately twenty nutrients, manufacturers add back four synthetic nutrients: niacin (vitamin B_3), reduced iron, thiamine mononitrate (synthetic vitamin B_1), and riboflavin (vitamin B_2). These meager synthetic nutrient additives are not digested or absorbed by your body as readily as whole food sources. Oh, and did you notice they bleached it, too? Awesome, thanks.
- High-fructose corn syrup is one of the most perniciously fattening substances on the planet. This genetically modified, sickly sweet syrup is associated with skyrocketing blood sugar, obesity, type 2 diabetes, B-vitamin deficiency, hyperactivity, tooth decay, and indigestion, among many other maladies.
- Dough conditioners can cause mineral deficiencies, and many processed breads include the same chemical that gives yoga mats their texture. I lived in an apartment above a Subway in college, and after smelling the noxious fumes of whatever substance was baking downstairs every morning, I can tell you that it's not bread. Subway was recently exposed by a blogger for using the same chemical used to

form little bubbles in yoga mats to give their breads a similar bubbly texture. A report from my friends at the Environmental Working Group found that the compound, azodicarbonamide, is used in close to five hundred food products, from Pillsbury Dinner Rolls to Little Debbie products to Wonder Bread.

- Ammonium sulfate may cause mouth ulcers, nausea, and kidney and liver problems.
- Sodium stearoyl lactylate may be corn, milk, peanut, or soy based, and may cause high blood pressure, kidney disturbances, and water retention.
- Brown sugar is frequently refined white sugar with molasses or artificial chemicals for coloring added. Sugar is sugar—stay away.
- Mono- and diglycerides are known to cause allergic reactions.
- Partially hydrogenated soybean oil is associated with obesity, heart disease, breast and colon cancers, atherosclerosis, elevated cholesterol, and reduced sperm count.

To your body, many of these substances are novel and unrecognizable as food. Before you buy anything in a package, take a look at the ingredients on the back and make sure that it's made with real food. Ask yourself: Where did these ingredients come from—a farm or a lab? As Joan Gussow quipped, "I trust cows more than chemists."

Pesticides in Our Corn

Here's a rhetorical question: Why is the same company that manufactured Agent Orange, a highly toxic herbicide responsible for poisoning millions since its use in the Vietnam War, making our corn?

Incredibly, scientists at this company, Monsanto, have discovered a way to genetically splice a *toxic pesticide* into the very DNA of corn itself. This genetically modified grain is known as "Bt [*Bacillus thuringiensis*] corn," and it already accounts for 88 percent of all corn grown in the United States. That means that when you eat this corn, or any product that contains corn-derived ingredients (such as high-fructose corn syrup, corn oil, or maltodextrin), you're swallowing a toxic pesticide.

Monsanto insists that Bt corn is perfectly safe for humans. Here's why that bothers me: Our bodies are less a single "human" organism than a high-level ecosystem comprising many different cells, bacteria, and organelles. In fact, you may be surprised to learn that nearly nine out of ten of the cells in and on your body right now are not technically "human," but belong to tiny bacteria that we've only just begun to study (you'll learn more about them on page 53).

Now, the toxic Bt pesticide that is engineered into the majority of corn grown in America is designed to rupture the stomach of any unfortunate bug that swallows it, causing death. We know that nine out of ten cells in our bodies are made of little bugs, necessary for our health. But wait a minute. . . . Isn't the Bt toxin designed to kill little bugs by making their stomachs explode?

And mind you, none of this genetic modification is done for the sake of your health and well-being, but for the profits of the same company that invented Agent Orange. Monsanto isn't exactly known for the safety of their products. How could we possibly trust them with our food?

In the United States, Big Food doesn't even have to tell you which foods contain this genetically altered corn on the label or whether it was used to feed the animals you're eating. No wonder Europe won't import our food. Even China, the country known for feeding poultry feces to its farmed fish, banned our meat and much of our processed food. We can do better.

I don't know about you, but I thought corn was perfectly fine before chemical companies started turning vegetables into toxic weapons. Growing up, my brothers and I would always fight over the first sign of sweet, crunchy sugar corn when harvest season came.

I would never tell you to deprive yourself of real, fresh corn straight off the stalk—but I will recommend you go organic. Organic certification lets you know that your corn is free of intentional GMOs and grown without petroleum-based chemical fertilizer.

HOW TO AVOID GENETICALLY MODIFIED FOODS

The genetic engineering of foods is a contentious topic. Perhaps one day we'll actually develop GMO foods that are beneficial for our health, but we're not there yet. The truth is that foods today aren't genetically modified for the sake of your health, but to cut costs and increase profits for Big Food. While GMOs are banned in many other countries due to concerns about their safety for human consumption, the United States doesn't even require food manufacturers to disclose whether their products *contain* GMO ingredients. However, a growing number of consumer-conscious food manufacturers—usually organic—now display the "Non-GMO Verified" seal on their products. Avoid the products below and on the following page and seek organic and non-GMO verified options when you can.

Common Products That Contain GMOs

KELLOGG'S: Rice Krispies • Corn Flakes • Frosted Flakes • Special K • Apple Jacks • All-Bran • Corn Pops • Crispix • Froot Loops • Frosted Mini-Wheats • Raisin Bran • Pop-Tarts • Eggo Waffles • MorningStar Farms Vegan Veggie Burgers • MorningStar Farms Chik'n Nuggets • MorningStar Farms Veggie Sausage • Keebler Chips Deluxe • Famous Amos Cookies • Carr's Table Water Crackers

KRAFT/NABISCO: Chips Ahoy! Cookies • Capri Sun • Boca Burgers • Cheez Whiz • Cool Whip • Corn Nuts • Crystal Light • Country Time • Honey Maid Graham Crackers • Jell-O • Kool-Aid • Kraft Singles • Lunchables • Maxwell House Coffee • Miracle Whip • Fig Newtons • Oreos • Oscar Mayer • Philadelphia Cream Cheese • Planters Nuts • Polly-O • Ritz Crackers • SnackWell's • Teddy Grahams • Triscuits • Velveeta • Wheat Thins

FRITO-LAY: Lay's Potato Chips · Doritos · Tostitos · Cheetos · Fritos · Sun Chips · Cracker Jack · Rold Gold Pretzels · Ruffles · Munchies · Stacy's Pita Chips · Smartfood Popcorn

QUAKER OATS: Quaker Oats Oatmeal · Life Cereal · Oat Bran · Quick Oats · Instant Oatmeal · Natural Granola · Chewy Granola Bars · Rice Cakes · Grits · Wheat Germ

NESTLÉ: Nesquik · Butterfinger · Crunch Bars · Kit Kat · Nescafé · Buitoni · Lean Cuisine · Hot Pockets · Stouffer's · Coffee-Mate · Carnation · Juicy Juice · Nestea · Dreyer's · Häagen-Dazs · Nestlé Ice Cream

CAMPBELL'S SOUP: Condensed Soups · Chunky Soup · Select Harvest · Healthy Request · Pace · Pepperidge Farm · Prego · Swanson · V8

COMMON GMO INGREDIENTS

1. **Soy:** soy flour, lecithin, soy protein isolates and concentrates (protein shakes). May contain GMO soy derivatives: vitamin E supplements, tofu, cereals, veggie burgers, soy sausages, tamari, soy sauce, chips, ice cream, frozen yogurt, infant formula, sauces, protein powder, margarine, soy cheese, crackers, breads, cookies, chocolates, candy, fried foods, shampoo, bubble bath, cosmetics, enriched flours and pastas.

2. **Corn:** corn flour, cornstarch, corn oil, corn sweeteners, syrups. Products that may contain GMO corn derivatives: vitamin C supplements, corn chips, candy, ice cream, infant formula, salad dressings, tomato sauces, bread, cookies, cereals, baking powder, alcohol, vanilla, margarine, soy sauce, soda, fried foods, powdered sugar, enriched flours and pastas.

3. **Cotton:** oil, fabrics. Products that may contain GMO cotton derivatives: clothes, linens, chips, peanut butter, crackers, cookies.

4. **Canola oil.** Products that may contain GMO canola: processed foods, chips,

crackers, cereal, snack bars, frozen foods, canned soups, candy, bread, hummus, oil blends.

5. **Sugar beets:** sugar. Products that may contain GMO sugar beets: any product that doesn't specify "cane sugar" but just "sugar" on ingredients, cookies, cakes, ice cream, donuts, baking mixes, candy, juice, yogurt.

6. **Alfalfa:** used to fatten livestock. Products that may contain GMO alfalfa: all types of conventionally raised meat, pork, poultry, eggs, and dairy.

7. **Aspartame:** artificial sweetener. Products that may contain aspartame: diet soft drinks, diet foods, yogurt, gum.

8. **Dairy:** rBGH growth hormone. Products that may contain GMO rBGH: all conventionally raised dairy products: milk, cheese, butter, yogurt, ice cream, and whey.

According to the Non-GMO Project, the highest-risk genetically modified crops include:

Sugar beets (approx. 95% of U.S. crop in 2010)

Soy (approx. 94% of U.S. crop in 2011)

Canola (approx. 90% of U.S. crop)

Cotton (approx. 90% of U.S. crop in 2011)

Corn (approx. 88% of U.S. crop in 2011)

Alfalfa (first planting 2011)

Zucchini and yellow summer squash (approx. 25,000 acres)

Papaya (most of Hawaiian crop; approx. 988 acres)

Avoid Processed Grains

We've known for hundreds of years that carbs make us fat, but the fat-free craze drowned out our common sense. Any food that contains finely ground flour—whether from wheat, rice, or other grains—will stimulate an undesirable jump in blood sugar. The more finely ground the flour and glycemic the carb source, the more quickly your blood sugar will rise. We enjoy wild, black, brown, or red rice or sprouted ancient grains in the evening a few nights a week. But when fat loss is the goal, cutting back on grains is a time-tested trick to drop weight fast.

The proof is in the pudding. You can ask any rancher in Texas:

How do you fatten a cow?
Feed it grains.

How do you fatten a human?
Feed it grains.

Humor me for a moment. What is your favorite part of a hamburger? The meat, the bacon, the gooey cheese, grilled onion, tomato, and seasonings, right? And how about pizza? Most people don't even eat the crust unless it's stuffed with cheese. These days, bread, dough, and other starches are often little more than vehicles for their toppings. Flour isn't delicious in and of itself. Flour relies on added flavor, usually in the form of salt, sugar, or fat, to make most products palatable. Have you ever swallowed a spoonful of white flour? Ick.

DID DON DRAPER INVENT BETTY CROCKER?

While researching the history of food processing for this book, I discovered that the affable "Betty Crocker" was never in fact a real person but a personality carefully engineered by a marketing team. In 1921, the new star of food marketing, Betty Crocker, was invented by the advertising department at Washburn Crosby (which later became General Mills) as part of a calculated campaign to drive American women to the company's expanding catalogue of convenience foods. For nearly a century, on television, radio, and magazine advertisements, Betty has promoted processed grain-based products with catchy slogans like "grand time savers" to appeal to busy moms. Responsible for moving millions of products made from cheap, shelf-stable ingredients and sold for stiff markups, Betty Crocker is one of the most profitable commercial characters of the twentieth century.

Do you need to cut out bread, pasta, grains, and other starches forever? No way! I'd never deprive anyone of a few treats during holidays and special occasions. But that's just it: They're treats, not dietary staples. Indulgences, not health foods. If you do choose to eat grains, enjoy them in moderate quantities (ideally on exercise days) and go for whole grains like brown rice, buckwheat, or quinoa to limit digestive stress from high-glycemic domesticated modern grains. Sandwiches and pasta dishes are often convenient but grain-heavy, so look at the recipe section for hearty fat-burning meals that will help you reach your goals.

With few exceptions, including an occasional bite or two of fresh-baked bread as a special treat, I prefer life without wheat, GMO corn, and other modern grains. Once you drop them, it's like health starts to happen automatically.

The Sordid Story of Soy

For decades, we've endured marketing spin about how soy is a health food. But, like many other processed foods, soy isn't ubiquitous because it's healthy—it's being pushed because it's profitable. In reality, processed soy is no health food.

The soybean was an unpopular crop until food manufacturers intent on creating cheap vegetable oils successfully persuaded the government to subsidize it. After processing the soybean to oil, the manufacturers were left with an industrial waste product—isolated soy protein. In order to boost profits, food manufacturers took the waste soy protein isolate and effectively created a market for it.

Now a veritable cash cow, soy is present in roughly seven out of ten foods on grocery store shelves in the form of soy lecithin, soybean oil, vegetable oil, texturized vegetable protein, soy flour, soy protein isolate, and more. Since nearly all the soy produced in the United States and Canada is genetically modified and contaminated with pesticides, it's best to avoid any food with soy products or by-products in the ingredients. Be careful—soy can be found in everything from protein shakes and bars to veggie burgers and imitation cheese. Go for real cheese instead. And if you don't dodge soy for the sake of your health, do it for taste. Compare a soy burger with vegan cheese product to a grass-fed burger with a sharp aged cheddar, and you'll see what I mean.

Processed soy acts as a goitrogen that disrupts your body's absorption of iodine and reduces thyroid function. Your thyroid regulates your metabolism, so when it falters, you gain weight and encounter a slew of other negative effects. Soy is also packed with antinutrients including phytates, enzyme inhibitors that block mineral absorption in the digestive tract. Soy contains a variety of toxic chemicals that cannot be fully metabolized by the body unless it undergoes extensive fermentation, which doesn't happen when soy shows up in processed food products. If you choose to eat soy, go organic and stick to its uses in traditional fermented foods such as miso, tempeh, or natural soy sauce (tamari).

The False Promise of Processed Oil

Packed with trans fats, pesticides, and chemical solvents, industrial seed and vegetable oils have been making us fat and diseased for decades. Deep down, we all know that real old-fashioned butter gives us something that fake butter just can't—no matter how hard Big Food tries to convince us otherwise. (Yes, we *can* believe the off-white, tasteless, odorless whipped vegetable spread hocked by Fabio is not butter.) Because the natural fats we crave, like real butter from cows raised on pastures, aren't just more delicious, they're also much better for us than the fats we see on commercials.

While real butter is still made by simply churning milk, much like your grandmother may have, modern vegetable oil processing looks more like a meth lab than Grandma's kitchen.

Genetically modified canola oil, for example, is obtained through a combination of high-temperature mechanical pressing and solvent extraction. Traces of the solvent (usually the petroleum-derived hexane) remain in the oil even after extensive processing. Canola oil is subjected to caustic refining, bleaching, and degumming—all of which involve high temperatures and/or chemicals of questionable safety. And since canola oil easily becomes rancid and foul-smelling when exposed to oxygen and high temperatures, it must be deodorized.

Before canola reaches the supermarket shelves, the deodorization process removes a large portion of the beneficial omega-3 fatty acids and turns them into trans fats, which are linked to heart disease and cancer. Since these trans fats occur in trace amounts, food manufacturers are not required to disclose them on their labels.

By the way, did you know that the word *canola* was invented by food marketers, too? The real name of the canola plant is rapeseed, which marketers assumed wouldn't sell well for obvious reasons. Instead, Big Food renamed rapeseed oil "canola," an amalgam of "oil" and "Canada," where the seed was popularized and continues to be grown today.

WHAT THE NUTRITION FACTS DON'T TELL YOU

Watch out for deceptive marketing statements like these on product labels:

- Fat-Free!
- Reduced Fat!
- Sugar-Free!
- No Added Sugar!
- Diet!

What these phrases often mean in practical terms:

- Fat-free, but packed with sugar and chemicals to compensate for the lack of flavor.
- Reduced fat, but increased carbohydrates and stratospheric glycemic index.
- Sugar-free. Artificial everything else.
- No added sugar . . . because the insane amount of "naturally occurring" sugars are enough to give you type 2 diabetes.

- "Diet" food, because it is literally watered down to "reduce" calories. Oh, and it causes brain tumors in lab rats.

Be careful of statements like these as well:

- All Natural Ingredients!
- 100% Natural!
- No Preservatives!
- No Artificial Preservatives!
- No Artificial Ingredients!

Statements like these mean next to nothing. Snake venom is 100 percent natural, too, but I wouldn't spread it on my toast.

Whenever a food claims to be good for you because it *doesn't* have something in it, be wary. For decades, "sugar-free" has translated to "known carcinogens that kind of resemble sugar"; "fat-free" to "tastes like cardboard"; and "natural flavors" to "may or may not contain the anal secretions of beavers" (see page 32). Remember, you want your food to be nutrient-dense, which means no junk calories (or "calorie-free" chemicals).

The healthiest foods are often the simplest ones, so aim for the fewest ingredients possible. For example, if you're picking out almond butter, look for almonds and perhaps salt on the label, but put down the jar if it has added sugars, processed oils, emulsifiers, preservatives, or anything else. These additives make products cheaper and last longer on the shelf, but they will also make you fat and sick.

WHY COUNTING CALORIES IS A WASTE OF YOUR TIME

FDA loopholes allow food manufacturers to manipulate the nutrition facts by omitting chemicals, additives, trans fats, and other substances from their labels. Nutrition facts are often doctored to make it appear that you're eating fewer calories than you actually are. Not only is it impossible to gauge your exact meal-to-meal calorie and macronutrient requirements, but trying to will drive you crazy.

If you're trying to lose weight by counting calories, you might want to reconsider. Does how much you eat have an impact on your weight? Sort of—fat loss doesn't depend on *how many* calories you eat, but on *which* calories you eat and *when*. Not only that, but because food manufacturers can manipulate the calorie counts listed on labels, most people drastically underestimate the number of calories they consume.

Even if the calorie counts on packaged food were accurate, the idea that your body "burns off" calories equally regardless of food source oversimplifies the matter. If you listen to Big Food, they'll tell you that drinking 100 calories of soda is the metabolic equivalent of eating a can of tuna fish. I don't buy it. Our bodies aren't like the incinerators they use in labs, burning calories one at a time—our bodies are incredibly complicated, intelligent, and self-regulating systems that want to be healthy. When you eat real food and trust your senses, you'll never have to count a calorie again.

BEWARE OF FOOD THAT DOESN'T SPOIL

If a food product can last on the shelves for extended periods of time, take a good look at its ingredients. Have you heard about the fourteen-year-old hamburger from McDonald's that still hasn't gone bad? Or the ice cream sandwich from Walmart that never melts, even on a hot day? If Mother Nature (and Father Time) won't even touch it, how confident are you that your body will recognize a bar of processed chemicals as food?

Real food gives your body the signals it needs to know that you just ate, while processed food encourages overeating, food intolerance, and eventually most of the diseases of the modern world. If your food doesn't go bad, or if ants refuse to eat it, drop that corn dog.

The Negative Effects of Industrial Food Processing

- As much as 90 percent of phytonutrients, which radically improve health and fight disease, are destroyed.
- The physical properties of foods are chemically altered in a manner that renders them dangerous. For example, homogenization and high-temperature pasteurization alter the fat molecules in milk, giving them properties that contribute to inflammation and heart disease.
- Minerals and natural cofactors are stripped from the food. Synthetic vitamins are often added into the flour to compensate, but synthetics are often not adequately digested since they lack the natural substances present in real food to increase bioavailability.
- Calories are concentrated in unnatural ways. For example, corn is processed into high-fructose corn syrup, which contains concentrated sugar devoid of fiber—a combination impossible to find in nature.

THE APPETITE ENHANCER
HIDDEN IN MORE THAN 700 FOODS

Many of us know that monosodium glutamate (MSG) is used as a chemical additive in most processed and fast foods. But do you know why?

MSG is a chemical used frequently by Big Food to *stimulate your appetite* and fool your brain into making low-quality food taste better than it actually does. But not only does MSG make you hungry, it also makes subjects predictably *gain fat* in the lab: Scientists frequently inject lab rats with MSG to literally *induce* obesity. Be careful—free glutamate, the damaging substance in MSG, can be hidden in almost anything, including sauces, condiments, jerky, chips, candy, chewing gum, and drinks.

Aside from appearing as monosodium glutamate, or MSG, this hunger-inducing substance often hides within the following more marketing-friendly ingredients:

- Autolyzed plant protein
- Autolyzed yeast
- Calcium caseinate
- Gelatin
- Glutamate
- Glutamic acid
- Hydrolyzed plant protein (HPP)
- Hydrolyzed vegetable protein (HVP)
- Monopotassium glutamate
- Senomyx (wheat extract labeled as "artificial flavor")
- Sodium caseinate
- Spices
- Textured protein
- Vegetable protein extract
- Yeast extract

No wonder we're all hungry. Avoid all packaged food with MSG or any of these ingredients on the label. When eating out, order your sauce and dressing on the side, as most are contaminated with MSG and other appetite-enhancing chemical additives.

DON'T BE DUPED BY "NATURAL" FLAVORS

The chemical flavoring industry is worth billions of dollars, practicing its furtive magic just off the New Jersey Turnpike. Although most consumers don't know much about the chemical flavoring business or its wily ways, chemicals are largely responsible for giving processed foods the smells and tastes that hijack your senses and create the illusion of real food. For example, you can sniff test tubes in the lab that smell exactly like your favorite burger, fries, or shake. Creepy.

Distinctions between artificial and natural flavors are relatively meaningless, based more on how the flavor has been manufactured than on the chemicals it actually contains. If you see "natural flavor" or "artificial flavor" on a label, you're holding a chemical soup.

For example, a typical artificial flavoring like the one in a McDonald's strawberry milkshake may contain some or all of the following ingredients:

amyl acetate, amyl butyrate, amyl valerate, anethol, anisyl formate, benzyl acetate, benzyl isobutyrate, butyric acid, cinnamyl isobutyrate, cinnamyl valerate, cognac essential oil, diacetyl, dipropyl ketone, ethyl acetate, ethyl amyl ketone, ethyl butyrate, ethyl cinnamate, ethyl heptanoate, ethyl heptylate, ethyl lactate, ethyl methylphenylglycidate, ethyl nitrate, ethyl propionate, ethyl valerate, heliotropin, hydroxyphenyl-2-butanone (10% solution in alcohol), a-ionone, isobutyl anthranilate, isobutyl butyrate, lemon essential oil, maltol, 4-methylacetophenone, methyl anthranilate, methyl benzoate, methyl cinnamate, methyl heptine carbonate, methyl naphthyl ketone, methyl salicylate, mint essential oil, neroli essential oil, nerolin, neryl isobutyrate, orris butter, phenethyl alcohol, rose, rum ether, g-undecalactone, vanillin, and solvent.

I'd rather have a strawberry, thanks.

Think you're better off eating foods with "natural flavor"? Chew on this: Secretions from the anal glands of beavers produce a bitter, smelly, orange-brown substance known as castoreum that is used extensively in raspberry and vanilla flavoring. It's legally labeled as "natural flavoring."

This is what happens when you trust food manufacturers, my friends. I hope you like beaver butt.

Honestly, I'm not as worried about the natural flavors made from crushed beetles or the rear ends of rodents; I'm much more concerned about the chemicals that trick your brain into thinking processed food actually tastes like anything good. Unlike real food, since chemicals can be owned as property, these newfangled substances are sped through production and often remain untested for human safety.

In some cases, natural flavors—like citrus—are actually made from the thing they are trying to approximate, but usually they're made in the lab. With few exceptions, I avoid all artificial flavors and most natural flavors, especially vanilla and raspberry. Flavors should come from plants, not smoking cauldrons in labs off the New Jersey Turnpike.

IF YOU'RE ADDICTED TO FOOD, IT'S NOT YOUR FAULT

If you've ever been caught knuckle-deep in a bag of Fritos, you're not alone. Processed food is engineered to hijack your brain to tell you that you're hungry when you're not.

If you take a bite of something and immediately crave more, drop it. That craving is indication that the pleasure centers of your brain have been hijacked. This is what most processed foods are designed to do, since craving more makes you eat and purchase more of the product, which means higher profits for Big Food. Obviously, there's a conflict of interest between your health and their boardroom meetings, and I think you know to which side the executives with $400 haircuts lean. In my time as a consultant, I worked with several of the biggest food manufacturers in the world, and I can tell you that many of the executives don't even feed their own products to their children. I asked one executive why, and he huffed, "Because they're all chemicals!"

WHY WE'RE ADDICTED TO SUGAR

Can't kick your sugar habit? You're not alone. We're wired to love sugar, and Big Food knows it. Big Food uses cheap, concentrated sugar (or, more often, high-fructose corn syrup) in almost everything because sweetness makes even bad food taste reasonably good. The sugar in our food adds up quickly, leaving many of us overweight and addicted. Today, just by including processed and restaurant foods in our diets, we're being exposed to more sugar in a year than our ancestors would have seen in their entire lifetimes.

One hundred years ago, we consumed 4 pounds of sugar a year. Fifty years ago, we bumped it up to 12 pounds per year. Today, the U.S. Department of Agriculture reports that the average American consumes more than *152 pounds of sugar a year*. While we once ate minimally processed sugars like honey, molasses, and cane sugar, the vast majority of our sugar today comes in the form of processed high-fructose corn syrup and genetically engineered sugar beets.

Sugar is one of the most addictive substances on the planet. The sweet tooth is a vicious cycle that starts with eating sugar and ends (or doesn't end) with craving more sugar. But here's my promise: If you start whittling down the amount of sweet stuff you consume, your cravings will slowly but surely disappear. If you can get the sugar monkey off your back, you may never have to worry about your weight again. The less you cave, the less you crave.

As a rule, I do my best to avoid any packaged food with more than 3 to 5 grams of sugar per serving (or per bottle, if it's a drink). Be careful—Big Food knows that sugar on the label stops consumers from buying, so often the serving size you see on the label is much smaller than what any normal human being would eat or drink in one sitting. This is designed to make it seem like the food is less bad for you than it actually is. Look carefully at the number of servings in the package or bottle and keep the total sugar below 5 grams.

Hidden sugars are everywhere, especially in beverages and packaged, processed foods. Be vigilant. It doesn't matter what name it goes by—glucose, crystalline fructose, cane sugar, agave nectar—it's all sugar, and it will all cause you to store fat instead of burn it. Also, remember that anything ending in "-ose" is typically a form of sugar, as in high-fruct*ose* corn syrup, malt*ose*, dextr*ose*, and sucral*ose*, to name a few. And if you see something sweet with low or no sugar, make sure to look at the label to ensure that Big Food didn't add in any artificial sweeteners (aka "nasty chemicals") to compensate.

Don't worry—you won't have to go without sweet things when you go Wild. Alyson and I eat a treat or two most nights, and many of our favorite homemade desserts are included in this book. Try them yourself on pages 250 to 269.

HOW TO IDENTIFY HIDDEN SUGAR IN YOUR FOOD

Food manufacturers often hide sugar under more marketing-friendly terms such as "cane sugar," "crystalline fructose," or "brown rice syrup," but it's all the same once it crosses your lips. Spotting refined sugar in packaged food can be a harrowing task—you have to be a real ingredient sleuth to decipher the sugar code—but knowing some of the most common names for hidden sugar is a good place to start.

- Barley malt
- Brown rice syrup
- Brown sugar
- Cane syrup
- Confectioners' sugar
- Corn syrup
- Crystalline
- Date sugar
- Dextran
- Dextrose
- Diastase
- Diastatic malt
- Ethyl maltol
- Fructose
- Fruit juice concentrate
- Galactose
- Glucose
- Glucose solids
- Granulated sugar
- Grape sugar
- High-fructose corn syrup
- Invert sugar
- Lactose
- Malt syrup
- Maltodextrin
- Maltose
- Mannitol
- Raw sugar
- Refiner's syrup
- Sorbitol
- Sorghum syrup
- Sucrose
- Turbinado sugar
- White grape juice concentrate

If you're eating out and you taste a sauce, dressing, or dish that seems sweet, it's likely packed with sugar or an artificial sweetener. Be careful—ignorance isn't bliss when nutrition is concerned. If something tastes too sweet, it's usually not worth finishing.

LIQUID SUGAR: SODA, SPORTS DRINKS, AND FRUIT JUICE

For many, the consumption of liquid calories is the single factor that means the difference between burning fat and storing it on a daily basis. Surprisingly, it's not just soda that destroys diets. Sports drinks, sweetened teas, and fruit juice can be just as catastrophic to your progress.

Packaged juice is a lot less natural than it appears. Although it's labeled as "fresh-squeezed 100% orange juice," for example, large juice manufacturers like Tropicana and Minute Maid store their juice inside giant vats for months on end, often in the belly of shipping tankers. Processing removes oxygen from the juice to aid in preservation, but the flavor goes with it. To compensate for the lack of flavor in their juice, Big Food contracts artificial chemical companies to synthesize fragrances to make your orange juice appear to smell and taste like real oranges. The same chemical fragrances that make perfume, laundry detergent, and household cleaners smell like citrus.

As Alfred E. Neuman, the buck-toothed, red-haired star of *MAD Magazine*, mused, "We are living in a world today where lemonade is made from artificial flavors and furniture polish is made from real lemons."

Not only does the industrial juicing process destroy flavor and most nutrients and antioxidants from the juice, but processing also strips the fruit of its natural fiber. When you eat fruit and vegetables whole, the natural fiber slows the absorption of fructose and other natural sugars into the bloodstream and prevents spikes in blood sugar. Remove the fiber and you have a fattening beverage indeed. The processed fruit juice you find in the supermarket has been shown to increase the risk of diabetes, and a high intake of fruit juice has been linked to childhood obesity.

If you really like fruit juice, have a few sips, but don't try to fill up on it or drink it for the sake of health—that's just fancy juice bars' way of overcharging you for a sugar bomb. Go for a whole piece of fruit or a green smoothie instead (see page 112).

Why Artificial Sweeteners Don't Count as Calories

One of the best strategies for cultivating vibrant health throughout your life is to know where your food comes from. But have you ever wondered about what an artificial sweetener actually is? Aspartame (NutraSweet) was discovered in the 1980s after the new substance was accidentally licked off the finger of a scientist who was trying to synthesize a new antiulcer drug. Sucralose (Splenda) is no better—it was discovered by two lab students while experimenting with a new type of *chlorinated pesticide.* Oops . . . I mean, yum!

Before you're enchanted by the suspiciously low calorie or carb count on the nutrition label of a packaged food, keep in mind that the only reason zero-calorie artificial sweeteners don't count as calories or carbs is because they're not technically food—they're chemicals. But don't be deceived—these substances have side effects (remember Olestra, which caused "anal leakage" in thousands of unsuspecting dieters?). While Big Food invents proprietary artificial sweeteners to make a quick buck, remember that many artificial sweeteners marketed to us, like saccharin, are eventually exposed as what they really are: carcinogenic chemical compounds that have no business being called food.

So How Do We Satisfy Our Sweet Tooth?

When you eat something sweet, do your best to make sure some amount of nutrients come along with it. Fresh fruit is a nutrient-dense and convenient treat, whether eaten whole, dried, or blended with other ingredients to sweeten baked goods (as we do in some of our dessert recipes). Minimally processed plant-based sweeteners like pure maple syrup and raw coconut nectar (if you can, get it raw and local) contain trace minerals, making them good options for sweetening baked goods, beverages, and treats. Other flavorful sweeteners we use in moderation are coconut palm sugar, brown cane sugar, and blackstrap molasses.

Our favorite low-carb sweetener is the dried leaf of the stevia plant. Organic extracts of stevia can also work well in a pinch, but avoid processed "stevia" sweeteners. For example, Truvia, which is "made from stevia" and purports to be an "all-natural sweetener," goes through forty-two steps of processing to make it four hundred times sweeter than sugar. Sounds like a processed food to me. Instead, order the dried, crushed stevia leaf online or grow it yourself.

HOW BEBAC AND MOKOLO DROPPED 170 POUNDS

After a twenty-one-year-old male gorilla named Brooks died of heart failure in 2005 at the Cleveland Metroparks Zoo, biologists decided to investigate why their gorillas suffer from the same afflictions as humans in much of the developed world.

Although obesity is almost unheard of in wild animals, many creatures get fat and sick as soon as they're caged. From a young age, zoo gorillas show evidence of high blood pressure, high cholesterol and triglyceride levels, fibrosis of the heart, and obesity. In captivity, more than one-third of gorillas die of heart disease, much like modern humans.

Interestingly, before poor Brooks's heart stopped, his diet included bucketfuls of vitamin-rich biscuits that were specially formulated by nutritionists to meet the precise dietary needs of gorillas. Apparently, nutritionists have some work to do.

To see if they would have better luck with a more "natural" diet, the biologists decided to feed two surviving gorillas, Mokolo and Bebac, foods closer to what they would find in the wild. From that day forth, zookeepers wheeled out 10 pounds of fibrous vegetables including dandelion greens, romaine lettuce, endive, alfalfa, green beans, flaxseeds, and a multivitamin hidden in half a mashed banana for good measure.

Although Mokolo and Bebac consume about twice as many calories on their "wild" diet, the two gorillas dropped nearly 65 pounds each in the first year and now weigh in the range of their wild counterparts. But it's not just gorillas that benefit from going wild.

Many pet owners find that the weight, health, and vitality of their furry friends improves when fed their native, raw diet. We feed our Labrador, Bailey, raw meaty bones, scraps, and off-cuts of meat as often as we can, and she has more mojo than we know what to do with. See page 316 for tips on how to feed your pets Wild.

"BUT IF PROCESSED FOOD WERE SO DANGEROUS, SOMEONE WOULD HAVE TOLD ME!"

I'm telling you. We all want to believe that omnipresent regulatory agencies with their legions of scientists protect us from the profiteers in Big Food, or at least that chemical companies and food manufacturers act responsibly in the interest of public health.

Big Food execs work in an environment where profits and shareholders come first, not your health. After suffering through more boardroom meetings than I'd care to remember in my time as a consultant, I know for a fact that most processed food manufacturers won't go out of their way to tell you anything that might hurt their bottom line. They want you to buy their food, not be suspicious of it. But our sense of security is misplaced.

Big Food is expected to police itself, which it does just about as well as Wall Street. Unfortunately, regulators and advocacy groups—even if they do have your best interests at heart—are years behind Big Food, which can churn out newfangled chemicals and invent foodstuffs with incredible efficiency and speed to make a quick buck.

A century ago, four out of ten of us were farming. Today, farmers number four in *one hundred* and most work on large-scale petro-chemical-fueled monocrops like GMO corn, canola, and soy—a landscape that would have been utterly unrecognizable as a farm to previous generations that believed a good harvest came from working *with* the land, not against it.

This information is not meant to inspire paranoia or conspiracy theories. The people who run Big Food aren't evil, just shortsighted and often irresponsible with our health. As long as you limit your exposure, it's quite likely that the effects of all of these fake foods and foreign substances will be minimal. Do the best you can.

Remember: Your body is a biochemical marvel. It can squeeze every last bit of nutrition out of any substance remotely resembling food. Your body can literally turn Twinkies into fingernails. With mystical powers like that, is it really so hard to believe this simple, straightforward idea: that you can burn fat if you eat the foods our bodies are adapted to eat, and break a sweat from time to time? There is hope!

The takeaway? Real food—natural plants and animals that we have been consuming safely for thousands of generations—is always a safer choice than processed food. The closer you can get a food to its source, the better. Read the ingredients, take the extra step to find farm-fresh food, and meet the people who get dirt under their fingernails to make sure you have a hearty meal on your dinner table. Taking the time and effort to understand where your food comes from may be uncomfortable when you realize that some of it isn't as healthy as you once might have believed, but it's one of the most rewarding things you can ever do for your health and well-being.

PART II

The Wild Body

WHAT WONDERFUL GENES YOU HAVE

Most of us are "getting old" too soon and settling for far less energy and vitality than we deserve. Through instinct, animals stay lean and vital in the wild despite eating as they please when food is available. With a little bit of practice, you can do the same. In this chapter, you'll learn how to tweak your lifestyle and habits to make your Wild genes thrive.

We once thought that we were shackled to "bad genes"—the ones that steal our youth, cripple our bodies, and bum us out every time the doctors talk about them. But research is clear—lifestyle factors like how you eat, where you live, and how you move are each inputs of information your body analyzes to turn certain genes on and off. Any look at a "before and after" fat-loss picture reveals that the "after" often looks like a different person, with well-formed muscles, tight and clear skin, and improved posture. Your genes know how to thrive, too, and you can drive your body to adapt to remarkable health with careful tweaking to your lifestyle.

Epi-genetics is a cutting-edge science that demonstrates that the air you breathe, food you eat, way you move, and even the thoughts you entertain can reprogram your genes for better or worse. You are endowed with a genetic program 3.5 billion years in the making that knows how to build a healthy body. The code is there. But in the modern world, the ancient biological systems once designed to help us thrive can work against us.

The turbocharged, polluted, high-tech world we live in is a far cry from what our Stone Age genetics were expecting, and we're suffering as a result. We didn't always settle for a diagnosis of diabetes, cancer, or heart disease before our time. These diseases of the industrial world are not rooted in genetic inevitabilities but self-inflicted conditions that are a direct result of how we eat and the way we live. "Domesticated" bodies are overfed yet undernourished, sedentary but stressed, and confronted with an environment that is increasingly polluting our air, water, earth, and food.

Once upon a time, all humans were "wild" and nomadic hunter-gatherers. Before the industrial revolution, cities, and agriculture, everything was wild, native, and organic. This is how your body was, and is still, designed to live. But instead of fleeing terrifying beasts that want to eat us for lunch, now we need to use all the willpower and energy we can muster to dodge food all day.

Our bodies haven't adapted to the intentionally addictive products of Big Food and the environment of drive-thru convenience that comes along with it. Molten chocolate cakes don't exist in nature, nor do Slurpees or deep-fried ice cream; the sheer amount of sugar in these gut bombs would have been nearly impossible for our ancestors to obtain in the natural world. For instance, you'd need to down 3 pounds of carrots for the sugar equivalent of one bottle of Coke. Modern food products play to—and take advantage of—our instinct to binge on sweets designed to fatten us up in preparation for the meager times ahead.

The main philosophy of *The Wild Diet* is that the closer we can get to the environment our genes expect—the world of our ancestors—the more our bodies will thrive. Animals that eat their native diet in their natural habitat enjoy lives free of the diseases of modern civilization. But for better or worse, we don't live in the same world as our ancestors. The utopian wilderness our genes expect doesn't exist where most of us live but can still be found in camping trips and outdoor adventures. Thankfully, while industrial progress has left us with an increasingly unnatural world, it has also provided tools to fight back. In comes modern technology.

HOW TO LIVE WILD IN A WORLD OF TECH: A CASE STUDY

These days, most of us can't go out to forage for berries on the prairie or butcher our own wild boar. So to help explain how you can apply the back-to-roots principles of living Wild, I figure I might as well tell you precisely what's happening right now.

As I type this sentence, I'm soaking up the afternoon sun that peeks in through the live oak tree outside my window. My watch tells me that I slept like a rock last night. It's also tracking my movement, temperature, perspiration, heart rate, and sleep—uploading everything wirelessly from my wrist to the Cloud. This allows me to see how changes in my behavior, mind-set, and activity affect my biology. I'm barefoot, haven't eaten a meal in nearly twenty-four hours (don't worry, I feel terrific), and I'm wearing prescription lenses that block blue light to help regulate my circadian rhythm and reduce iStrain from my iMac. . . .*

Whenever I get stuck, I take a break to unplug and clear my head by avoiding visual, auditory, and other sensory distractions. In fact, I composed a few passages of this book while "floating" in a sensory deprivation tank, but I wrote most of it outside or in view of the window in daylight hours while fasting. By delaying my large meals until later in the day, I channel my energy to productive work throughout the day and save my feasting (and food coma) for the evening hours.

I do my best work in the woods, taking breaks for a hike with the dog, conquering a mountain on the bike, or howling old bluegrass songs where there's no one around to hear me. While I may edit and hone my work on machines, I do the vast majority of thinking when I'm on adventures in the wilderness, never without my notebook and a good pen.

*In case you were wondering how much of a nerd I am, I'm glad to have saved you the trouble. There's even a fitness tracker on my dog.

Later in this part, you will learn how to upgrade your health, productivity, and performance using what I call *holistic* biohacking. If you think of Western medicine as getting a patient from "sick" to normal, think of holistic biohacking as bringing your body from "normal" to "super-normal" by optimizing your lifestyle for health and performance. But first, let's talk about sex.

Like pretty snowflakes, we are all biochemically unique. Depending on your sex, genetics, body type, age, activity level, hormones, brain, rhythm, gut bacteria, enzymes, metabolism, and many other factors, the exact same diet will have different results for you than for your significant other, next-door neighbor, sibling, or even your identical twin.

You probably have an annoying friend or family member who never seems to gain a pound despite eating whatever they want, whenever they want. Good for them. But before you get envious, know that the genetic freaks with perpetual six-packs and see-through skin are also the first to starve in a famine. Variability in a population increases the likelihood of survival of the species as a whole. And that's good news for everyone.

HE SHED, SHE SHED: HOW MEN AND WOMEN BURN FAT DIFFERENTLY

Body Composition

Women are genetically designed to have a lower percentage of muscle and more body fat than men, principally to support the biological processes of pregnancy and childbirth. Because women naturally have less muscle than men, they typically have lower basal metabolic rates. This means that men, with a higher percentage of muscle, require more calories than women of comparable weight. Additionally, men are taller on average than women and require more daily calories to maintain their size.

Hormones

Women are naturally predisposed to store and retain more fat due to higher levels of estrogen, a hormone that works to keep the fat on the female body in preparation for pregnancy. Men, on the other hand, have twenty to thirty times more testosterone than the average woman, which often leads to lower body fat and increased muscle mass. This disparity in testosterone, the male sex hormone, is largely responsible for differences between men and women in total body fat percentage, fat distribution, and muscle mass. There are athletic trade-offs as well—men tend to be more muscular and women more flexible due to differences in genetics, hormones, and bone structure.

Fat Storage

Women typically store fat in their thighs, hips, and limbs, known as "peripheral" fat, and beneath the skin, which is called "subcutaneous" fat. Men tend to store more body fat in the upper body and within the body cavity, which is called "visceral" or intra-abdominal fat. Although all body fat is chemically similar, where it's stored on the body makes a significant difference in how hazardous it is to your health. While the female body tends to store the less-damaging peripheral fat underneath the skin, men tend to store damaging visceral fat that accumulates beneath muscles and surrounds organs. This often takes the form of the dreaded "beer belly."

Beer bellies aren't just unsightly, they're downright dangerous. The visceral fat that wraps around organs and forms beer bellies drastically increases the risk of diabetes, hypertension, sleep apnea, impotence, cancer, heart attack, and stroke. In fact, regardless of overall weight, men with waists exceeding 40 inches have double the death rate of those with normal waist circumference. Fortunately, hiding beneath every set of love handles and every beer belly there is a six-pack. We're going to find yours.

Muscle Gains

Many women hesitate to incorporate weight training into their weekly routines because they believe it will lead to brutish, hulk-like muscles. Unless you're taking growth hormones, testosterone, or steroids, that won't happen to you. The female body does not naturally have sufficient levels of hormones to achieve anything close to "bodybuilder" size. Trust me—you have nothing to worry about. My petite wife, Alyson, impresses onlookers at the gym with heavy dead lifts, squats, and swings and has never been slimmer or stronger.

Protein Consumption

Men generally carry higher muscle mass and lower body fat than women, so they tend to need more protein to maintain their size. That said, most people do not eat enough protein for optimal health; this is especially true for women. Meat is not a "man's" food. To support the biological processes of ovulation, menstruation, and pregnancy, some nutrients that are only found in animal foods are arguably even more critical for women's health. If you prefer not to eat meat, do your best to get protein from nuts, seeds, legumes, leafy greens, and whole grains. See "The Wild Diet for Vegetarians and Vegans" on page 312 for more.

Rate of Fat Loss

You may have noticed that while women often cut calories and exercise constantly with sluggish results, some men are mysteriously able to shed pounds seemingly without effort. This is not an illusion: Due to differences in hormones, metabolism, and body composition, males do tend to lose fat a bit more quickly while female bodies fight to hold on to it. Most of these sex differences stem from the fact that female hormones readily store extra fat to prepare a woman's body for the significant energy demands of ovulation, pregnancy, lactation, and childbirth.

If you're petite, you may lose weight more slowly than those who are larger. As such, pay attention to improvements in body composition rather than strict weight loss by the numbers. But there are some advantages to being smaller—even a small amount of weight loss will be quite evident on a small frame.

For both men and women, it is important not to measure success by looking at the scale but by how you look in the mirror, the way you feel in clothes, and/or by body fat percentage. Muscle weighs more than fat, water weight fluctuates according to a variety of factors, and weighing yourself constantly will drive you bananas. I've gained and lost 5 to 10 pounds in the same day on many occasions, none of which have anything to do with my love handles. Forget the scale and measure your progress by how you look and feel instead. Watching the scale won't help you lose fat more quickly, but watching what you eat will.

FAT-LOSS TIPS

For Women

INDULGENCE IS IMPORTANT, BUT SO IS MODERATION

What foods truly bring you pleasure? What foods could you eat less of? What foods do you eat to pointless excess? The pleasure comes in the first few bites of food—anything more is unnecessary and upsets the balance of your body. It is far more important and satisfying to eat small amounts of many tasty foods than enormous portions of one or two. You can really enjoy a little bit of anything as a treat.

LEARN THE ART OF BALANCE

Balancing your meals is an art learned with practice. If you have an extra glass of wine, then skip the cheese. If you have a rich lunch, have a light dinner. "Overdoing it" should always be followed by an active effort to restore balance. If it's easier, think of your nutrition in weeks, not days. Eating a vegetable or a protein every meal is a good guideline, but it's unnecessarily prescriptive. If you find that you don't have enough access to vegetables one day and eat several extra servings of protein, that's fine. On the next day, prioritize fibrous green veggies to maintain balance.

EMBRACE THE RULE OF QUALITY OVER QUANTITY

Most Americans are accustomed to eating very low-quality food. When you replace junk substitutes with the real thing, you immediately realize that less is more. Savoring one single piece of real chocolate is far more satisfying than eating a dozen Hershey's bars (which, oddly, contain more GMO corn than real chocolate). Go for the good stuff—you deserve it.

FASTING MAY BE MORE EFFECTIVE FOR MEN THAN WOMEN

In the next section, we'll cover my cyclical approach to eating, which I call "fasting and feasting." While the hormonal environment in the male body is relatively consistent, the fluctuating hormones in a woman's body are easily disrupted. While fasting works well for some women, fasting too much can stress the adrenals and cause your hormones to rebel. Adrenal burnout comes quickly when you combine hormetic stressors like exercise and fasting, especially if you're not sleeping well or you're emotionally drained. Listen to your body—if you find that going without a meal works well for you, know that there are many benefits to doing so. If not, plan ahead and make sure you have a steady source of healthy food that's always ready when hunger strikes—like nuts, veggies, fruit, and the always-convenient leftovers.

For Men

TESTOSTERONE—GET SOME

If you're experiencing symptoms such as decreased sex drive, erectile dysfunction, memory problems, or depressed mood, low testosterone may be to blame. Testosterone plays a critical role in sexual and reproductive function, muscle mass, hair growth, bone density, and more. But a man's production of testosterone begins to decline around age thirty and continues to do so as he ages.

As a man gets older, he tends to lose muscle mass and gain fat, largely due to a natural reduction in the body's production of testosterone and growth hormone. Since fatty tissue doesn't require the same amount of energy to maintain lean muscle, he gains weight over time even if his diet remains consistent. While women put weight on their breasts, hips, and limbs, men store fat around the gut, where it circulates through the liver, causing metabolic problems like diabetes. This extra fat puts you at risk of cancer, heart attack, hypertension, and sleep apnea and can also affect your sex life.

What if one nut could increase your metabolism, raise your testosterone, and boost your sex drive? Say hello to your new friend, the Brazil nut. High in healthy fat, protein, and trace minerals, Brazil nuts are one of the highest dietary sources of selenium, an essential trace mineral and potent antioxidant. Selenium boosts testosterone levels in men and improves sperm production and motility. Brazil nuts are also rich in the amino acid arginine, which increases levels of blood to the genitals. That's right—in the supermarket, nature's Viagra is found in the "nut" section.

TROUBLE IN THE BEDROOM?

If you've ever had trouble getting your mojo workin', you're not alone. A recent study found that about 49 percent of men ages forty to seventy-nine with high blood pressure had erectile dysfunction. Another study, published in the *Journal of Urology*, found that 68 percent of men with high blood pressure had some degree of erectile dysfunction. For 45 percent of the men, it was considered severe.

While the ephemeral diagnoses of high blood pressure can be easy to ignore or deny, impotence gets a man's attention. Did you know that impotence isn't just a problem with your erectile capabilities but actually one of the most obvious symptoms of high blood pressure, elevated triglycerides, and the initial stages of heart disease?

High blood pressure prevents the arteries that carry blood into the penis from fully dilating, while the smooth muscle in the penis loses its ability to relax. As a result, the body fails to send enough blood into the penis to make it erect. For that reason and many others, you don't want high blood pressure.

Can't I Just Pop a Pill for That?

If you watch the commercials during football games—you know the ones, with the good-looking silver-haired man in his Mustang and a hot trophy wife sitting shotgun—you'd think that taking drugs for sexual dysfunction is fashionable. But many prescription drugs work against each other, fixing one problem but breaking something else. For example, commonly prescribed medications that treat high blood pressure—like diuretics and beta-blockers—actually *cause* erectile dysfunction, and statins can decrease production of testosterone.

If you want to improve your performance in the bedroom, get your diet in line and engage in high-intensity interval training and/or strength training. By balancing insulin and boosting growth hormone, fasting can also help normalize blood pressure. Spare yourself the embarrassing trip to the doctor and an expensive prescription by eating Wild and committing to high-intensity workouts to bulk up and lean down as quickly as possible.

BE A REAL MAN AND COMMIT

The male body seems to get away with more overeating, laziness, and misbehavior than the female body. I've seen men achieve the impossible—losing 20 pounds in a week, dropping down to a skeletal 3 percent body fat in less than a month eating mostly fat, and fast for weeks without losing muscle or strength. As long as they eat clean and exercise consistently, most men tend to have an easier time losing fat and building muscle than women. The problem is, women tend to pay more attention to their bodies, so their level of commitment tends to be higher.

I know it's not "cool" for a man to care about his "diet," but if you can't do it for yourself, do it for your family and friends who care about you and want to keep you around for a long time. The better your health now, the more years in your life and life in your years. When you commit to eating right and staying in shape, you'll have more time with the people you love.

"But my friends will make fun of me for being on a diet!"

Maybe, but they'll also start coming to you for fitness advice when you're the only one in the group with a six-pack.

YOUR MICROBIOME: THE HUMAN ECOSYSTEM

Humans are more of an "ecosystem" than a single organism. Believe it or not, the human digestive tract is home to a dizzying quantity of tiny gut bugs (bacteria) that outnumber human cells ten to one. These bacteria are storehouses for an enormous amount of genetic information—genes that are switched on and off depending on the health of your microbiome, how you exercise, your diet, stress, how much sugar you eat, and much more.

The quantity and quality of your gut flora play an essential role in how you digest your food and how well you are able to obtain nutrients from it. Gut bacteria predigest your food, provide immune protection, and even release neurotransmitters that affect your behavior and mood (some refer to the gut as your "second brain"). Let's meet the two main categories of bacteria, the good guys and the bad guys:

- Probiotic (good) bacteria aid digestion, release nutrients, and protect the digestive system against dangerous pathogens. Fiber and raw fermented food feed good bacteria. Traditional methods of food fermentation yield positive probiotic bacteria that are readily introduced into your digestive tract. Our favorite fermented foods that you might find fizzing on our counter include kimchi, sauerkraut, yogurt, kefir, and kombucha.
- Pathogenic (bad) bacteria invade the body, steal nutrients, and release toxins into the bloodstream. Sugar feeds the bad bacteria, or "sugar bugs," the bad guys. Fasting and eating low carb starves "sugar bugs" of their main fuel source, and eating probiotic-rich foods and vegetable fiber helps to heal your gut and expel pathogenic bacteria.

The old saying "you are what you eat" is true, but it's incomplete. Your body can't access the energy in food the second it crosses your lips—you must digest and metabolize the food first. You have to disassemble your food before it's "reassembled" as part of your body or eliminated as waste. You aren't what you eat, you're what you *absorb* and assimilate. Since the gut and liver alter nutrients before they enter the bloodstream, the nutritional content of the food (what it says on the label) is fundamentally different from the nutrients and energy that are absorbed by your cells.

The types of bacteria living in and on your body also dictate whether you store fat or burn it as fuel. Lab studies have shown that the wrong species of bacteria in mice can make them gain fat no matter what they eat. We're just beginning to understand how these bacteria affect our own biology, but suffice it to say that I do my best to be good to my gut.

Just like you eat and excrete nutrients, bacteria do, too. While the bad bugs (pathogenic bacteria) excrete toxins and other substances that can disrupt metabolic processes, good bugs (probiotics) release vitamins and nutrients into your bloodstream. Bad bugs thrive on sugar, and good bugs thrive on fiber. Make sure you feed the right ones.

ANTIBIOTICS, CANONS, AND MOSQUITOS

With many of us popping antibiotics like candy, it's important to note that taking an antibiotic kills off not just the bad bacteria but the good bacteria in your gut as well. When you think about the literal meaning of anti-biotics (anti-life), that starts to make sense. Take antibiotics with caution, and make sure you use them only when absolutely necessary. If you do take an antibiotic, eat extra fermented, probiotic foods and round it out with a soil-based probiotic supplement to get your gut back on track. While prescriptions can clearly be useful and, at times, lifesaving tools, pills are also very easy to abuse.

The average American age forty-five and older is on four different prescription medications, a number I'd argue is far too high. Not only are synthetic drugs expensive, but they also cause side effects, steal nutrients, and interact unpredictably within the body. When I started using food as a tool to heal, I noticed that the symptoms I used drugs to treat—high blood pressure, insomnia, nagging colds and viruses, joint pain, allergies, and more—resolved themselves without pill-popping. I noticed another benefit of going wild—the several hundred dollars a month once spent on prescriptions were delightfully redirected to artisanal cheese, pâté, aged prosciutto, and the occasional bold Cabernet.

Be Good to Your Gut

In these days of fake food and broken guts, food intolerances and sensitivities are incredibly common. Many people do not realize that their unknown, undiagnosed food allergies and intolerances—primarily to processed grains, legumes, and dairy—are responsible for their weight gain, inefficient digestion, bloating, skin problems, allergies, and other health issues. Despite individual variance in food sensitivity and allergy, nearly everyone can benefit from eating more fresh, nutrient-dense vegetables.

Processed foods damage the gut, while most real, whole foods help to heal it. The Wild Diet helps heal "leaky gut" and other afflictions by encouraging consumption of plant and fruit fiber (which determines the amount and type of bacteria that thrive in your system), adding regular fermented food to your diet, and creating an environment that allows probiotic bacteria to thrive. Sugar bugs, be gone!

We almost always have something fizzing, bubbling, or growing on the counter—kombucha, sourdough, sauerkraut, sprouting seeds, and more. My friend and fellow author Tucker Max taught me this trick: If you want to improve the probiotic punch of store-bought kombucha, twist the cap and let it sit on the counter for a few days. The good bacteria in the bottle will go straight to work digesting the residual sugars, which will leave you with an authentic low-sugar fermented drink without the weeks of attention it usually takes to make kombucha from scratch.

The Cyclical Rhythm of Fasting and Feasting

The concept of time doesn't play a factor in most diets. But failing to address *when* we eat misses a critical dimension, one that could be the difference between vibrant health and unshakable sickness.

Against the relentless onslaught of advertising that taunts our deep-seated, primal urge to eat as often as we can, willpower isn't enough. Every thirty seconds, most of us are interrupted by a boisterous distraction that demands our gustatory attention:

"Quarter-Pound Hamburger for 99 cents!"

"Pizza! Pizza!"

"Hungry? Grab a Snickers."

Unlike our ancestors, who spent all day chasing a beast and all evening enjoying it, the smells, sights, and sizzles of food nag at us 24/7. In a world where everyone is eating all the time, it's difficult to know when we should actually eat.

As it turns out, three square meals a day—breakfast, lunch, and dinner—is arbitrary, more a cultural artifact than a biological necessity. The modern man isn't just eating *more* than he ever has but—critically—*more often* than he ever has. Eating from dawn to dusk gives our bodies a steady stream of glucose, damaging in excess. Without a break from the taxing requirements of digestion, most of our population is faced with insulin resistance, weight gain, and disease.

"Fasting and Feasting" is what I call a rhythm of meal timing that maximizes the hormonal benefits of under- and overeating. While skipping just the occasional meal can be beneficial, cycling periods of fasting (usually in the morning) and feasting (usually at night) can aid detoxification, encourage fat burning, and improve immune function. Fasting and feasting isn't meant to be dogmatic—it's simply the concept that your body thrives by following a cyclical approach to eating and digestion.

By one definition, fasting means "to abstain from all food." But it also means "to eat sparingly, or of certain types of foods." For the most part, I'm talking about the latter, less draconian definition. In the same way that our muscles and bodies recover from plenty of rest, wouldn't it hold that our digestive system would benefit from an occasional break from food?

Fasting Is Good for You

If you could put the mental, physical, and spiritual benefits of fasting in a pill, you would make billions. The many benefits of fasting include:

- Promoting human growth hormone production, which helps your body burn fat, build muscle, and slow the aging process
- Normalizing insulin sensitivity, which prevents chronic disease like diabetes, heart disease, and even cancer
- Normalizing ghrelin levels, also known as "the hunger hormone"
- Decreasing triglyceride levels
- Reducing inflammation and reducing free radical damage

While most nutritionists argue that we eat too much, I argue that we simply eat too *often*. By undereating most of the day and filling up at night, most people also find that they eat significantly less food (and save money) once they start fasting.

Let's dig a little deeper.

Calorie Restriction and Cyclical Undereating

Since the 1930s, animal studies have been telling us that restricting calories improves health and longevity. Until recently, we believed that it was necessary to "starve yourself" to reap the benefits. But you can actually trim your waistline, improve your biomarkers of health, and increase your longevity without the pain, suffering, and hunger that comes along with restriction. Fasting works, too, but since it's difficult for Big Food to profit from people going without their food, most of the benefits of skipping meals don't make it into common wisdom.

There's a monumental difference between "common" and "normal," however. Today, more than 67 percent of us in the United States are overweight or obese. Being overweight is common. But it's not normal. Fasting, on the other hand, is historically quite normal but isn't common in a world abundant with drive-thrus, meal-replacement shakes, and "eating 6+ times a day is healthy" dogmatism. For millions of people across the world, regular fasting is commonplace and has been part of spiritual practice for thousands of years. But before that, fasting was simply a way of life.

With no storable grains, and few other foods that stayed fresh for very long, most of our ancestors experienced both feast and famine on a regular basis. When game was scarce, seasons changed, or the pickings were slim, hunter-gatherers did without. To reap the full rewards of the Wild lifestyle, you might consider going without occasionally, too.

Antiaging Effects of Fasting

We've known for many years that eating less increases life-span in humans and animals, but "starving yourself" doesn't appear to be gaining much traction. Thousands of studies have shown that when animals are placed on a calorie-restricted diet, they invariably outlive their frequently fed counterparts. The longest-living and most disease-free cultures on the planet eat significantly less than the average American.

If you're over the age of thirty, and especially if you lead a sedentary lifestyle, you've likely entered a phase known as somatopause, or age-related growth hormone deficiency. Natural production of growth hormone declines beginning in our twenties, leading to a reduction in lean body mass and bone mineral density and an increase in body fat—especially abdominal fat. As growth hormone declines over time, you begin to look and feel older.

Here's the good news: Fasting sets in motion a hormonal chain of events that not only burns fat but also protects hard-earned muscle. After approximately sixteen to twenty-four hours in a fasted state, our bodies release a massive surge of growth hormone. One study showed that while fasting for twenty-four hours, human growth hormone increased an average of 1,300 percent in women and nearly 2,000 percent in men. But be careful: Depending on your unique situation, many find that you do begin to lose muscle with fasts that are longer than twenty-four hours. Listen to your body and eat when you're hungry.

Another activity that can lead to a dramatic increase in growth hormone is high-intensity interval exercise like the 7-Minute Wild Workout (see pages 81 to 83). Combining fasting with high-intensity exercise can provide synergistic effects to boost growth hormone. In adulthood, the presence of growth hormone leads to a healthier body composition. Growth hormone:

- Keeps your body lean
- Increases synthesis of new protein tissues to promote muscle recovery and repair

- Decreases fat accumulation
- Strengthens bones
- Protects your organs from the decline that occurs with age
- Promotes healthy hair and nail growth
- Improves circulation
- Gives a more favorable cholesterol profile
- Decreases signs and symptoms of aging

Did I mention that fasting is free and you can start right now?

Breakfast: The Most Dangerous Meal of the Day

Would you eat donuts for a "healthy" breakfast? Believe it or not, most products marketed as heart-healthy "breakfast foods"—cereal, granola, oatmeal, bagels, yogurt, and muffins—pack more sugar than a deep-fried, sugar-coated Krispy Kreme donut. Some cereals are even packed with more processed sodium than a bag of potato chips.

Cereal is a shining example of a product that Big Food intentionally mislabels to make it appear "healthier" than it actually is. In an analysis of 1,556 popular cereals, researchers at the Environmental Working Group found that "97 percent of the most common class of cold cereals have labels that underestimate the amount of cereal people actually eat." Since the serving sizes on cereal labels are unrealistically small, many Americans unintentionally eat more than one "serving" in a single bowl.

Many popular cereals are packed with more sugar than a scoop of ice cream, a jelly donut, or a slice of chocolate cake. Honey Smacks contains more than 50 percent sugar, and Apple Jacks, Froot Loops, and Corn Pops all contain 12 grams of sugar and almost zero fiber in the paltry serving listed on the side of the box. For perspective, a glazed donut from Dunkin' Donuts contains 12 grams of sugar. Surprised?

When you look at the ingredients in cereal and donuts, you really don't see much of a difference. Donuts are made from processed flour, sugar, and industrial oil. Cereal is made from processed flour, sugar, and . . . industrial oil.

Here's why that's a problem: Nobody eats a donut for breakfast and thinks they're doing themselves a favor. But how many people eat cereal for breakfast (or dinner) and assume that it is good for them? Cereal and bagels got me through college, but I didn't know I was eating dessert for breakfast.

People who start their days with carb-y, high-glycemic foods like cereal, muffins, bagels, and fruit juice ignite a vicious cycle of hunger and snacking. The flood of insulin in the hours following breakfast leads to low energy, brain fog, and nagging cravings and hunger throughout the day.

As any endurance athlete or adventurer quickly learns, most of your energy comes not from what you eat for breakfast but from your dinner the night before. The more nourishing and substantial your evening feast, the more you can do or longer you can go without eating the next day. Eating the *right* breakfast can help regulate your blood sugar, but it's not actually burned for fuel that day. Since the body takes eight to sixteen hours to process your meals, the majority of each day's fuel comes from the dinner you ate the evening before. Eating your most substantial meal in the evening can help release endorphins, improve sleep quality, reduce next-day hunger, and provide energy to fuel activities the next morning.

When I began fasting regularly, I learned that I tend not to get hungry until I start eating. Hunger pangs and cravings pass quickly, usually dissipating after just a few minutes. Once you fast for a few hours, your body moves carbohydrates out of glycogen stores in your muscles and liver to provide energy to fuel your brain and hunger is reduced.

According to our circadian rhythm, melatonin rises after sundown to help us sleep, and cortisol—a stress hormone—rises in the morning hours to wake us up. If you eat in the morning when blood cortisol is high, however, high-glycemic carbs cause insulin to spike and decrease sensitivity to insulin. That's one of the reasons you might be starving a couple of hours after a big, carb-y breakfast. Eating from dawn to dusk, while it certainly works for some people (especially those who eat real food), can also provoke an insatiable urge to keep eating. How often have you stared at the clock, eager for the next mealtime? Frequent snacking trains your body to be hungry. Fasting does precisely the opposite.

The more you adapt to burning fat by eating fewer carbs and occasionally fasting, the less you think about food. When you can get through your day without the distraction of constant hunger, you can get a heck of a lot more done. Enjoy the energy that comes with digestion-free workdays as your peers look on in awe.

When you graze on frequent meals throughout the day, your body assumes that you live in a time of plenty and spends energy readily. A steady supply of glucose leads your cells to divide readily to perform bodily functions, store fat, and build muscle—you can think of this as "build" mode. Cell division is biologically expensive, however; research suggests that constant grazing may accelerate the aging process by decreasing the length of telomeres. Fasting, however, signals your cells that it's time to focus the body's energy on conserving, restoring, and repairing your body's internal machinery. You can think of fasting as "cleanse" mode, where your cells scavenge your body for free radicals, agents of disease, and damaged cells and recycles them to conserve energy. The trade-off is that too much fasting can stress the adrenals, so occasional luxurious feasting can actually help keep the body in balance.

HOW TO BEAT FALSE HUNGER

True hunger is generally experienced in the body and brain, not in the stomach. If you get light-headed or weak, or your workout suffers, you're probably fasting too much. It may take some practice, but once you reconnect with the feeling of true hunger, you can follow your body's lead and eat whenever the feeling strikes.

Whenever you get hungry, ask yourself:

- Am I thirsty? Drink water and cravings may subside.
- Have I had my fill of greens and fiber today? Go for a salad, veggies, or a green smoothie.
- Am I emotional or bored? Wait twenty minutes, go for a walk, or exercise.
- Did I drink alcohol recently? Your body is probably tricking you into thinking you're hungry because your insulin is out of whack.

- Have I eaten my fill of protein today? Grab some.
- Did I eat sugar, grains, fried food, or other "carbage"? Your insulin and blood sugar are unstable. You probably don't need more food. Wait it out.
- Have I exercised today? Try it and you might find you're not hungry anymore.
- Am I fasting too much? Go ahead and eat. Bonus if you make raw green veggies the first thing to hit your belly.

What If I Really Need Breakfast?

No problem. If you want to lose fat and you prefer not to fast, eat a light, low-carb, high-protein breakfast. If you like savory, farm-fresh eggs are tough to beat. A green smoothie or plain yogurt with nuts and berries is also a filling, nutritious, and convenient breakfast. But remember—eating too many carbs early in the day can make you feel sluggish because the insulin flood shifts your body to "rest and digest" mode, which is great for falling asleep at night but not great when it hits midday. To maximize fat loss, save your carbs (and insulin) until directly after your workout (to build muscle and refuel glycogen stores) and your evening meal. If you eat a particularly large or rich meal (or know you will for dinner), scale back the other meals to avoid overdoing it.

But if you find you are not hungry in the morning, there's no need to force it. Many people find that after their first few tries fasting, hunger doesn't come until you "flip the switch" by eating something.

FREE YOURSELF FROM FOOD

When I started taking fasting seriously, my energy and productivity doubled, I dropped fat while gaining muscle, and I was finally freed from the unrelenting hunger that plagued me for most of my life. Interestingly, I also learned that I don't tend to get hungry until whenever I choose to have my first meal, usually in the afternoon. Many of my listeners are surprised to learn that I record my weekly hour-long shows on the same day back-to-back, often eight or more without a meal. When I'm finished with work in the evening, I'm ready to *feast*.

But wait—why would you get more energy from eating less often? As anyone who's just polished off a slice of birthday cake knows, digestion takes energy. Bloating, brain fog, that banal, empty feeling where you just want to take a nap—this is "rest and digest" mode, when your body redirects the energy that otherwise would have been used to fuel the brain and body to try to make use of whatever the heck was in that corn dog. Ugh.

"WHAT'D YOU HAVE FOR LUNCH?"

When Alyson and I showed up at the photo shoot for the cover of the hardcover edition of this book at one thirty in the afternoon, my photographer asked cheerfully, "So, what'd you guys have for lunch?"

"We haven't really eaten yet, actually," Alyson replied.

The photographer turned to his wife and smiled. "And *that's* why they're so lean!"

Mentally, I enjoy the freedom that comes with eating later in the day. While everyone else is feverishly trying to figure out what the heck they should eat for their next meal, I'm sipping tea and thinking about something else. If I skip breakfast to get straight to my morning routine and plan for a larger meal later in the day, I find that I'm full of energy until the afternoon or evening without a substantial meal. This affords me an extra couple of hours a day during which I would have otherwise been finding, preparing, or eating breakfast, lunch, and snacks.

So, what do you do while everyone else is eating breakfast and lunch? Anything you want. All the time it normally takes you to find, prepare, and eat extraneous meals has just been transformed into 100 percent free time. If finding, preparing, and eating breakfast and lunch once took a total of two hours a day, that's what you've got. Enjoy that extra two hours to do whatever you please. Think about it . . . an extra two hours of free time every day for the rest of your life. Take that, *4-Hour Workweek*.

Here's how the Fasting and Feasting eating pattern stacks up against a standard American eating schedule.

STANDARD AMERICAN EATING PATTERN

MORNING	Meal 1	Breakfast
	Meal 2	Snack
MIDDAY	Meal 3	Lunch
	Meal 4	Afternoon snack
EVENING	Meal 5	Dinner (and dessert)
	Meal 6	Evening snack

Total: 6 meals. Time to find, prepare, and eat meals: 2 to 3 hours.

FASTING AND FEASTING

MORNING	Beverages	Water, coffee, tea, herbal tonics
MIDDAY	Meal 1	Raw veggies, fruits, nuts, and light snacks
EVENING	Meal 2	Glorious feast (and dessert)

Total: 2 meals. Time to find, prepare, and eat meals: 45 to 60 minutes.

The Fasting Phase: Foods to Eat During Daylight Hours

When I "fast" during the day, I don't always go without *all* calories. I start most mornings with heavy cream in my coffee (pure fat), and I might snack on raw nuts or veggies or sip on bone broth whenever it feels right. Most days, I prefer to eat at least one light meal before my evening feast, usually at midday or in the afternoon. One way I think about Fasting and Feasting is that I eat raw foods during the day and cooked meals at night. Since we spend as many days as we can hiking, mountain biking, or adventuring, we don't cook our first meal until we get back to base camp as the sun sets (a cooked feast is also great for morale). If I get real hunger during daylight hours, I eat light foods that won't steal too much energy for digestion—salads, green smoothies, or even raw vegetables like celery, cucumbers, or carrots for a snack.

Here are a few examples of low-calorie, low-carb, light foods I might eat during "fat-fasting":

- Raw green vegetables like cucumbers or celery
- Grass-fed butter, ghee, or cream (in coffee or melted on leftovers)
- Green smoothie
- Carrots
- Avocado
- Coconut
- Nuts
- Jerky
- Sardines
- Bone broth
- Bone marrow
- Soup
- Plain yogurt
- Raw cheese

While undereating during the fasting phase, drink plenty of water and enjoy as many naturally calorie-free drinks such as coffee, tea, and seltzer as you like. When you get hungry, eat freely from the snacks above, but do your best to save your largest meal until the evening feast.

Fasting on a Whim

If you're not hungry at mealtime or just can't find clean food, go ahead and skip a meal every once in a while. Just have a glass of water or an herbal tea. This often happens when I'm traveling, when I didn't plan to skip a meal but it just feels right anyway. Great! This temporary "fasting" will allow your body to burn fat and direct its energy to repair and recovery instead of digestion.

Fasted Exercise for Rapid Fat Loss

If you want to drop fat as quickly as possible, work out fasted. Research suggests that the effects of eating Wild and exercising in a fasted state are synergistic; eating low-carb boosts the body's responses to human growth hormone, while fasted exercise boosts its production. If you're looking to gain muscle, improve recovery, and upgrade performance, this is exactly what you want.

When Not to Fast

Fasting and Feasting is completely optional on the Wild Diet. Fasting is easy when life is good, but it doesn't work for everyone. If you're stressed, sleepless, or someone who burns through calories with reckless abandon, you don't need the added stressor of going without food, which can actually increase the risk of overtraining. If you feel dizzy, weak, or confused while fasting, it's time to eat. Food is fuel, so make sure you get enough. The first few times you try fasting, make sure you have plenty of healthy snacks ready when the going gets tough. Take it slow and let your body adapt.

Fasting isn't advisable during pregnancy, while nursing, if you're diabetic, or if you have a history of eating disorders. As mentioned earlier in this part, some women find that skipping meals can lead to weight gain, mood swings, disrupted sleep, and worse. You may find that skipping meals simply isn't for you. That's great—now you know that. If you feel differently in the future, go ahead and try it again to see if you feel the same way. But if going without food for part of the day truly makes you miserable, there's no need to force it.

Before you start fasting, I suggest that you avoid processed carbs, sugars, and starches for a few weeks and fill up on high-protein foods to let your body adapt to running on fat. Once the fat-burning mechanisms of your body are firing on all cylinders, you can learn to trust your hunger and appetite. In a healthy body, you can listen to your instincts and simply eat until you're full.

How to Break Your Fast: The Anabolic Effects of Feasting

If you're worried you'll waste away if you don't suck down a protein shake every two hours, don't be. When I started my experiments with fasting, I was afraid that I would get weak and all of my hard-earned muscles would fall off. But instead, I hit a personal best in my dead lift and gained 10 pounds of lean muscle while consistently skipping breakfast.

My approach to Fasting and Feasting involves eating a generous meal later in the day; usually in the afternoon between noon and three p.m., or whenever I get hungry. This tends to work out to sixteen to twenty hours a day of undereating—running on nothing but fat—and four to eight hours of feasting. When I can, I feast after an intense workout to maximize anabolism (a fancy word that means muscle building and repair).

Each fast concludes with the promise of a big anabolic payoff. To make the best of the surge of growth hormone after sixteen hours of fasting, work out during the last few hours of your fast. Your post-workout feast breaks the fast, and the circulating growth hormone acts to partition the nutrients from your meal to your glycogen stores and muscle fibers. It's natural to crave carbs following exercise because you burned through muscle and liver glycogen during your workout. Eat some, but make sure you go for natural options—such as sweet potatoes, bananas, whole-grain rice, dairy, or coconut water—instead of processed products marketed to athletes. Protein powders are convenient, easy choices for post-exercise feeding, but real fresh food like sweet potatoes, eggs, and dairy are usually better for you.

Fasting and Feasting can also be applied at the macro level by cycling your intake of food on a weekly or monthly basis. Since overeating sometimes happens naturally, I often treat vacations and holidays as an extended feasting phase. Like a bodybuilder in a "building phase," I exercise more frequently and with heavier weights than usual in an attempt to use the extra carbs and calories to grow muscle. When I return to my normal habits, I treat the following few days as a "cleansing" phase. To compensate for overeating during the feasting phase, I fast more often in the days after; drink plenty of teas, tonics, and liquids; and consume smaller meals, primarily green and fibrous vegetables.

Get Started Now: Fasting and Feasting Plan

How do you start? Simple. Tomorrow, make lunch your first meal. If you stop eating at eight p.m. and don't eat until noon the next day, that's sixteen hours of fasting—perfect for stimulating growth hormone, which boosts metabolism, builds muscle, and slows aging. The fact that you sleep through the majority of your fast makes it relatively painless.

If you've trained your body to expect food every two hours, then you might feel hungry the first few times you try fasting. But it will all be in your head. Running just on the fat stored in their bodies, most Americans could walk from New York to Florida without actually needing a bite to eat. Give yourself a week or two for your body to re-learn how to run on fat, and you'll find fasting gets easier.

Fasting shouldn't feel like *forcing* yourself not to eat food. While fasting, you're liberated from having to think about food so you can spend your energy elsewhere. That little voice that usually nags every few minutes, *"Hey, is it time to eat? I think it's time to eat!"* now has a response that works every time. "There's an epic feast coming tonight," you might say. "No need to bother me until then." After all, you have important things to do today.

The best day for your first fast is your day off, perhaps Sunday, so you won't fall prey to the stress of the workday. Do your best to get plenty of sleep and have a satisfying feast the night before your first fast to keep cortisol in check.

YOUR MENU:

9:00 a.m.—Fatty Coffee (page 249): 1 cup of coffee with 1 tablespoon heavy cream, coconut milk, butter, or other real-food fat

Noon—**Meal 1:** Giant salad with avocado, cucumber, and feta over mixed greens drizzled with olive oil and balsamic vinegar

6:00 p.m.—**Meal 2:** Beef Tenderloin with Buttered Onions, Horseradish, and Arugula (page 181)

7:00 p.m.—Dessert: Strawberries and real grass-fed whipped cream

If you get hungry between lunch and dinner, eat freely of the snacks listed beginning on page 305. Remember to drink plenty of water and spice it up with a bit of herbal tea or club soda with a slice of citrus if you're in the mood for a tasty drink. Good luck—I'll see you on the other side.

WATCH OUT—FASTING MIGHT MAKE YOU SUPERHUMAN

I don't really know how to explain it, but there is a fascinating phenomenon that often kicks in when people try fasting. Once you find that you *can* in fact go without food for some or most of the day with great energy, you ask yourself: "What else am I capable of?" That's where life gets interesting.

I'll offer my own example. In my first two years of regular fasting, I went from a struggling musician with a desk job to a multiple-award-winning talk show host, bestselling author, and millionaire at the reins of the hottest food app publisher in America. With the extra time, clarity, and confidence you get from fasting, you might find that the entire trajectory of your life changes. Get in touch at FatBurningMan.com and let me know how it goes.

RECALIBRATE YOUR CIRCADIAN RHYTHM

Have you ever spent all night looking at the ceiling, cursing yourself for not getting a wink of sleep? Me too. I was always a terrible sleeper, lucky to get six hours of restless sleep at most. I'd count hundreds of sheep, take drugs, write, have sex, perform full-body muscle relaxation, meditate, try breathing exercises—nothing seemed to work. Now I sleep like a baby—working on this book, I'm usually conked out by nine thirty p.m. What changed?

Nearly all organisms are programmed to honor cycles of light and dark. We call these cycles circadian rhythms. Our blinding and noisy world of electronics and artificial lights, many of which are bright enough to mimic the sun, upset these rhythms. When your biology is out of sync with your environment, a circadian "mismatch," you pay the price with disrupted sleep, agitation, digestive disorders, constipation, chronic fatigue, chronic cravings for sweets and carbs, fat gain, and decreased resistance to stress.

Your circadian rhythm affects your eating pattern, but few people realize that what you eat and when can recalibrate your circadian rhythm. Habitually eating too much in the morning and throughout the day works against our natural eating patterns and saps energy. Big, heavy, carb-filled meals put our bodies in "rest and digest" mode, when nutrients and energy are diverted to digestion.

Large feasts in the evening can help you fall straight to sleep, so it's best to save heavy meals and carbs until dinner if you want to maximize energy during the day. If you have trouble waking up or falling asleep, consider catching at least fifteen minutes of sunlight in the morning and avoid artificial lights after sundown to reset your circadian rhythm.

Contrary to popular belief, sleeping for eight hours at a time is not necessarily the best way to sleep for everyone. Sleeping this way popped up only within the last hundred years—post industrialization—when artificial lights made it possible to keep working after sunset. But before that, human beings slept more like animals: in two short segments—a long sleep just after dusk, followed by quiet waking time in the middle of the night, and then a return to bed for a morning nap. Don't be afraid to take naps or sleep in—we've been refreshing our bodies and brains with siestas for thousands of years.

When you fall asleep shortly after the natural darkness of the night and wake with the sunrise, without an alarm, feeling rested, you are in sync. If you're thinking that requires more time in your bed, you're right, and you're welcome. Like Benjamin Franklin said, "Early to bed, early to rise, makes a man healthy, wealthy, and wise."

THE BIG SECRET THE TABLOIDS
WON'T TELL YOU

Want to know how superstars, fitness models, and professional athletes stay so lean and become superhuman? They sleep. A lot.

No, it's not some sexy new thigh-sculpting machine, fat-blasting wonder drug, or superfood from a country you've never heard of. These specimens of mankind probably just sleep more than you. If you want to cure yourself of nearly any affliction known to man or feel like a rock star, you need more sleep. How do you know when you've had enough? Sleep until you reliably can wake up without an alarm (hopefully somewhere in the neighborhood of the sunrise).

Not only will getting a good night's sleep help to reduce your risk of disease, but it will improve your focus, sharpen your reflexes, and give you the energy you need to rock it. Remember that muscle isn't built in the gym—it recovers and grows while you sleep. Sleep and rest is also prime territory to burn fat. So be honest with yourself—is your four a.m. workout really improving your performance or just stressing you out? A simple rule: If you don't get solid sleep, don't overdo it in your workout. Sounds crazy, but if you exercise smart, you can get away with far less time sweating than you'd expect.

If you have trouble sleeping, try this:

- Get fifteen minutes of sunlight early in the day to reset your circadian rhythm.
- Eat a large feast after sundown and let your "rest and digest" mode trigger an early bedtime.
- Avoid artificial light and electronics after sundown (or use blue-blocking lenses).
- Drink chamomile or kava tea, natural plants that relax the body and mind, in the evening.
- Supplement 0.5 to 1 mg of melatonin after sundown.
- Carry an eye mask and earplugs in your overnight bag for noisy or bright environments.

- Use heavy, light-blocking shades in your bedroom.
- Avoid strenuous exercise in the hours before sleep.
- Keep your bedroom cool; most people sleep best at less than 70°F.
- Go to bed at the same time every night, even on the weekend, to avoid disrupting hormones.
- Avoid alcohol, which prevents the body from entering deep, restorative sleep (one or two drinks with dinner is fine).
- Meditate for ten minutes before bed to calm your mind.

PART III

Wild Movement

> **If you're not having fun, you're doing something wrong.**
>
> —*Groucho Marx*

The modern world seems like it's built to prevent us from using our bodies. Today, many of us spend the majority of our waking hours seated in front of a desk or steering wheel. Your body doesn't know quite what to make of this, given the fact that humans moved constantly for millennia. We've never *needed* to exercise—physical movement was simply a requirement of life.

Imagine a jaguar stalking silently through the jungle, muscles rippling under its coat. This beast is capable of exploding into action with blinding speed, but all that power is channeled into smooth, fluid, effortless movement—beautiful to watch. This is how humans are meant to move, too: with grace, power, and economy. For the vast majority of human existence, we spent all day moving: walking, running, pulling, pushing, and lifting. These lean, hard bodies—male and female—were required for work and survival.

One of the first Europeans to explore the American Southwest was Álvar Núñez Cabeza de Vaca. He lived among the Native Americans for eight years in the sixteenth century and witnessed their legendary strength and vigor firsthand. Impressed by their epic feats of athleticism during the hunt, he wrote: "The men were happy, generous, with amazing physical prowess. . . . One Native American ran down a buffalo on foot and killed it with his knife as he ran by its side. . . ." The natives were also notoriously difficult to kill: "Traversed by an arrow, he does not die but recovers from his wound. . . ." Cabeza de Vaca continued, "They go naked in the most burning sun, in winter they go out in early dawn to take a bath, breaking the ice with their body."

Our bodies are capable of much more than most of us realize. Remember this the next time you're dreading your workout or standing on the shore of a lake afraid it's too cold to jump in. Your body is meant to withstand hot and cold, and stimulating the biological machinery to adapt to the seasons is good for you. But don't worry—you don't need to live like Tarzan to get as lean and fit as a wild animal.

WHY GRINDING ON A TREADMILL IS NOT THE BEST WAY TO BURN FAT

The diet industry tells us that we need to "burn off" calories if we're to have any hope of dropping a few pounds. Trainers might tell you to spend an hour on an expensive machine that measures all the calories you burn off down to the last Tic-Tac. "Eat less and exercise more!" they declare.

But you don't need to grind it out on the StairMaster all day or powerlift with greased-up meatheads to get in shape. Exercise is not about "burning off" your burger or punishing yourself—it's about your well-being. To put calorie burning into perspective, you'd need sixty minutes on the treadmill to "burn off" the amount of calories in one Starbucks muffin. There's a better way.

In this chapter, you'll learn how to perform simple exercises that drive hormonal and metabolic changes to burn fat, build muscle, and improve performance. You will be amazed at how much you can achieve with a few short, intense bursts of exercise that take just minutes a week.

A "DOSE" OF EXERCISE

There's a common assumption that more exercise is better, but it isn't that simple. Some types of exercises are much more effective for fat loss, and they might not be the ones you think.

The best use of exercise isn't for burning off calories but for setting off a hormonal cascade in your body that results in an adaptive response. This process is called hormesis, which is a biological response to low doses of a stressor that improves the ability of the body to handle stressors in the future.

While homeostasis seeks to bring the body to a normal state, hormesis brings the body to a better-than-normal state. For example, when an athlete lifts weights, the stress of the heavy load damages the muscles by overloading them. The body reacts with inflammation and an immune response—in small doses, these otherwise problematic processes are beneficial to the body, as it uses inflammation and stress to rebuild and grow stronger. Whenever your body faces a challenge and you give it what it needs to recover, you come back bigger and better every time you push yourself.

Your body needs to be constantly challenged in order to become stronger and leaner. For most people, it takes a few weeks to adapt to a routine and reach the point of diminishing returns. Doing the same exercises over and over can cause burnout and repetitive stress injuries. Keeping your body guessing and unable to adapt by ensuring variety is part of your exercise routine. If you'd like to build and tone your muscle, prioritize strength-training sessions. If you want to lose fat quickly, prioritize interval training. Once you're strong enough to breeze through your workout, it's time to add to the weight and change it up.

WHY DO I *HAVE* TO EXERCISE?

You can accomplish a lot just by eating Wild. You'll burn fat, build lean muscle mass, and boost your metabolism. Bodybuilders often say that six-packs are carved by spoons—meaning that what you eat (and don't eat) will determine how much fat you carry—and they're right. If you want to drop fat, you need to eat right. But if you want to step it up a notch, you'll have to move your body. With an effective exercise plan, you can kick off a hormonal cascade that moves your physiology toward being lean. You can achieve spectacular fat loss and body composition with far less exercise than the fitness industry would lead you to believe. And it's not only possible but essential that you find exercises and activities that you love.

When someone asks for my secret to six-pack abs, I tell them that it's as much about how I live as how I train. Here's the truth:

I eat clean and fast several times a week. I spend most of the day with my core engaged—standing, moving, or sitting cross-legged. I schedule intense full-body workouts in my calendar and stick to them like I booked a flight.

Exercise isn't about your vanity; it's about your well-being. The flood of endorphins and other raw materials that your body releases during and immediately following exercise literally helps you get stronger and smarter.

An enormous amount of brainpower is dedicated to the countless feats of movement we achieve without even thinking about them. Recent science has shown that the brain can actually grow, adapt, rewire, and repurpose itself—this is known as neuroplasticity. Actively moving and training your body helps your brain *grow* and has been shown not just to improve your body but increase your intelligence as well. This mental and physical training is what allows amateurs to become Olympians, and it's not just their bodies but their brains that adapt to the incredible demands of the professional athlete.

THE POWER OF FULL-BODY, FUNCTIONAL MOVEMENT

There's a reason that Mickey trained Rocky for his fight against Apollo Creed by jumping rope, sprinting up stairs, and chasing chickens through the alley—each task takes an efficient nervous system, quick reflexes, and economical, balanced movement. In the cult wrestling classic *Vision Quest*, while Louden Swain's hopeless competitors train on pegboards and machines, the camera cuts to the freakish, undefeated farm boy adversary who's slogging up the bleachers in the pouring rain with a tree on his shoulders. That's functional movement, and you don't need fancy machines when you train like that.

When you work out, use your whole body. Studies have found that explosive full-body movements like squats, dead lifts, and pull-ups increase our anabolic hormones like growth hormone and testosterone while decreasing circulating cortisol, a stress hormone. On the flip side, isolated exercises like bicep curls aren't a great use of time if you want to lose fat. These one-muscle-at-a-time moves don't stimulate enough muscle fibers to build lean muscle or expend enough energy to maximize your calorie burn, and they lead to only incremental gains in the exact muscles you isolate. Whole-body exercises that target the large muscle groups in the legs and back are a better strategy for fat loss.

WHAT ABOUT MY AB ROLLER?

Despite what the late-night infomercials and checkout-aisle magazines tell you, ab-crunching, -rolling, and -shocking gadgets won't give you a six-pack, and doing traditional ab exercises such as crunches and sit-ups don't cause fat loss on your stomach any more than bicep curls would. The key to getting sculpted abs is to burn off the fat that covers them. This is best achieved by full-body movements that incorporate the large muscle groups—like squats, presses, dead lifts, pull-ups, and kettlebell swings—which set off a hormonal cascade to boost fat metabolism. Once your abs are visible, ab-targeted exercises like planks, crunches, bicycle kicks, and even pull-ups can increase definition.

Aim for balance in your movements to create symmetry in your body. For example, if you're stuck in one position for most of the day, do your best to exercise in the opposite position. If you spend most of the day crouched forward for your job, take on a sport like kayaking that incorporates a full range of motion to open up your back and shoulders. If you've done a few too many push-ups, make sure you strengthen the opposite muscles in your back with rows or another equal-and-opposite movement. (I'm actually writing this on the floor in a "Sphinx" position right now to stretch my back.)

These days, you can learn just about any exercise for free with a search on Google. To ensure you learn correct form for lifting heavy weights or high-intensity exercises, however, I suggest you find a well-respected trainer. Ask him or her to construct a proper high-intensity interval workout with a complementary full-body strength-training program tailored to your specific goals. There are a lot of bad trainers out there—ask friends, check reviews, and don't be afraid to shop around to find a trainer who will motivate you to achieve more than you could on your own.

Poor form leads to injury, and getting hurt will kill your progress. Learn the movement, start slowly, prioritize proper form, and reexamine your movements from time to time to ensure you're not getting sloppy. If a trainer isn't in your budget, spend five bucks and grab a jump rope. Jumping rope provides an awesome full-body workout that will tone you up quickly with minimal effort. And if you think jumping rope is for little girls, it's time to rewatch *Rocky*.

CASE STUDY: HOW TO LOSE FAT BY EXERCISING LESS

When I first studied the science that suggested I could exercise for just minutes a week and lose fat, I had to see it for myself. At the time, I was running 50 miles a week, often for several hours a day. After finishing in the top 3 percent of runners in my previous marathon, I assumed that I was in tip-top running shape. I figured that running less would make me slower and fatter. The results are far more interesting.

By switching from endurance to sprints, I gained 10 pounds, but I actually *lost* body fat! The muscle that came on from my new sprint routine combined with the fat loss increased definition and size in my shoulders and abs. My body regained healthy color and a more masculine shape, and my running speed and strength increased dramatically. I felt *tons* better. Even my face changed from hauntingly thin to healthy and full—all from exercising much *less*.

Have you ever noticed that most endurance athletes are rail-thin, pale, and look a little unhealthy? But what about athletes who are required to perform short bursts of maximum output, like sprinters, linebackers, soccer players, and wide receivers? They're lean and mean!

When it comes to getting lean and fit, your body responds to quality over quantity. Exercise is beneficial only up to a point, after which you start wasting muscle instead of building it, retaining fat instead of burning it, and flooding your body with stress hormones that throw your metabolism out of whack. This is known as overtraining.

If you're overtrained, your body doesn't know you are running a marathon or if you've just been run over by a truck. Your nervous system simply knows that it is experiencing trauma. So, your hormones go wacky, your fight/flight response is heightened, and your body pumps out stress hormones. For long-term training, fat loss, and health, this is all bad news. Because it's always trying to recover from what you just did to it and protecting itself from whatever might happen next, your befuddled body never has a chance to heal. Due to the presence of stress hormones, you readily store fat—the opposite of what you're hoping for when you're putting in all those miles. Give your body time to recover and it will reward you with improved performance and a leaner physique. Remember: You build muscle and burn fat while you sleep, not when you're in the gym.

If you live for endurance athletics like marathons and triathlons, more power to you. Finishing such an event is a tremendous accomplishment. But know that endurance exercise isn't the best solution to fat loss. Intensity trumps endurance when body composition is concerned, so don't skimp on intervals even if you are an endurance athlete. Besides, running is more fun when you pretend you're being chased by a tiger.

THE 7-MINUTE WILD WORKOUT

A word of caution: Intervals are extremely vigorous. If you are a beginner, get your doctor's clearance before attempting any type of high-intensity exercise such as high-intensity interval training.

Want more bang for your buck? If you're short on time, try a 7-minute Wild Workout. A Wild Workout session consists of 20 seconds of maximum output followed by

10 seconds of rest repeated 10 times without pausing for a total of 5 minutes. Each session begins with a 60-second warm-up and ends with a 60-second cooldown.

The Wild Workout results in unique changes in skeletal muscle and endurance capacity that were previously believed to require hours of exercise each week. While moderate aerobic exercise improves only aerobic systems, the interval training actually improves both anaerobic (intense, muscle-building) and aerobic (slower, oxygen-consuming) body systems.

If you want to look and feel like an athlete, the following workout will help you train more like one. This routine is based on science developed by the Japanese Olympic Speed Skating team in the 1970s, finding that a work session followed by even shorter periods of recovery dramatically improved speed, power, and performance as compared to endurance cardio.

Hill sprints are a fantastic interval workout for beginners and veterans alike. Steep inclines reduce impact on your joints and require more power from the large muscle groups in the legs. Give yourself 7 minutes, and you'll get more out of this workout than most people do in 2 hours on a treadmill.

All you have to do is find a hill with a steep incline and run as far and as fast as you can for 20 seconds—give it absolutely everything you've got. There are two alternating phases to the Wild Workout—a work phase and a recovery phase. For a 7-minute workout, you will perform 10 sets of 20-second sprints with 10 seconds of recovery between each set. It looks like this:

Warm-Up: 60 seconds of light cardio, mobility, and dynamic stretching.

Workout: 10 sets for a total of 5 minutes.

Work Phase: Sprint for 20 seconds as fast as you can without stopping.

Recovery Phase: Rest for 10 seconds. Catch your breath and get ready for the next round.

Cooldown: 60 seconds of light cardio, mobility, and dynamic stretching.

Before you begin, shake out your joints and get your juices flowing with a quick warm-up. To begin your workout, start your timer and sprint as fast as you can up the hill. After 20 seconds, take 10 seconds to catch your breath before your next sprint. You should be huffing and puffing as soon as your 5 minutes starts and completely out of juice by the end. The last few rounds should be almost impossible. Remember, you get out of exercise what you put in, so don't let that whiny voice that sometimes pops into your head psych you out of a great workout.

Don't have a hill for your workout? Any high-intensity exercise will do—sprinting, bicycle sprints, jump rope, jumping jacks, burpees, rowing, swimming, and anything else that gets your blood pumping. The 7-minute workout is a great place to start, but if your level of fitness requires more rest, go ahead and take it. When I'm without my timer, I often sprint at a slightly lower intensity for as long as a minute, counting in my head. I follow longer work intervals with more rest—if I sprint for a minute, then I rest for longer than 10 seconds. Feel free to use this workout as a template to customize as your fitness improves with more sets and shorter rest.

Everybody else loves to hate it, but my favorite full-body interval workout while traveling or limited on space and time is the infamous burpee. Professional athletes, CrossFit trainers, and elite military forces swear by the dreaded burpee, which just might be the ultimate full-body exercise. It's viciously efficient and uncompromisingly effective. You're probably sweating just by thinking about it. If you don't know what a burpee is, hold on to your hat.

HOW TO PERFORM A BURPEE

1. Begin in a squat position with hands on the floor in front of you (leapfrog position).
2. Kick your feet back, while simultaneously lowering yourself into the bottom portion of a push-up.
3. Return your feet to the squat position, while simultaneously pushing up with your arms (perform the push-up while returning your feet to the squat position).
4. Leap up as high as you can from the squat position and extend your arms above your head, reaching toward the ceiling.
5. Move as quickly as possible back to the first position.
6. Repeat. No wussing out.

STRENGTH WORKOUT

Regardless of your gender, if you want a sexy body, get your lift on and build some muscle. High performers focus on intensity, explosive movements, and muscle adaptation, not "face time" in the gym. If you want to burn fat, boost your metabolism, tone your muscles, and strengthen bone mass, then lifting weights is far more effective than cardio. Lifting heavy things increases lean muscle tissue, one of the body's most powerful mechanisms for burning fat. The more lean tissue you have, the more calories you burn, which increases your resting metabolic rate.

To maximize hormonal response, perform full-body exercises that stimulate as many muscles and expend as much energy as possible at the same time. My favorite full-body exercises include:

WARM-UP

- [ ] Jumping jacks
- [ ] Shadowboxing
- [ ] Dancing
- [ ] Jogging

BODY WEIGHT

- [ ] Sprint
- [ ] Squat
- [ ] Push-up
- [ ] Pull-up
- [ ] Burpee
- [ ] Handstand push-up

MINIMAL EQUIPMENT

- ☐ Kettlebell swing
- ☐ Jump rope
- ☐ Resistance band pulls

GYM EQUIPMENT

- ☐ Weighted squat
- ☐ Dead lift
- ☐ Row
- ☐ Bench press
- ☐ Leg press
- ☐ Lat pull-down

ABEL'S STRENGTH-TRAINING TIPS

Exercise your entire body during each workout—the legs, trunk, core, arms, and shoulders.

Focus on symmetry, form, and balance to avoid injury.

Lift heavy—use a weight that you can only lift 5 to 15 times before compromising form. If only lighter weights are available, focus on bursting into the movement and continue until exhaustion.

Use a steady cadence for each lift to eliminate momentum and ensure constant load.

Aim for 2 sets of 5 to 15 reps for each exercise. As soon as you can't make it through a movement with good form, it's time to stop and rest.

Rest at least 30 seconds between sets, longer for monster lifts with heavy weights like dead lifts and presses. You want to rest long enough for your muscles to recover enough to make it through your second set, but not so long that you start to cool down.

Aim to finish your workout in 45 minutes or less.

If building strength or size is the goal, overload your muscles with increasing weight. Once 10 to 15 reps can be performed with perfect form, increase the weight by 10 to 20 percent.

WHERE TO START?

If you're not ready for a high-intensity workout or monster lifts, that's okay. Everyone starts somewhere. Building the habit of moving your body on a regular basis is far more important than any short-term fitness goals, so know that the most important step is to consistently show up for your workout. Make the space for consistent exercise sessions or outdoor adventures in your schedule and stick to them like you booked a flight.

If you're out of shape, start with low-intensity aerobic exercise like walking and strength training. You can start interval training once your fitness level improves in the weeks ahead. Here's the good news if you're carrying extra weight: You have more muscle than you think, mostly in your legs and thighs to support your trunk. The muscles in your thighs are little fat-burning factories, and yours are likely already developed. Start with some squats and you'll have a huge head start on the skinny people.

WILD WORKOUT PROGRAM

1. Break a sweat every day.
2. Walk often, preferably outside in the sun at least once a day.
3. Complete one strength workout a week.
4. Complete one interval workout a week.
5. Rest at least one day a week.

I'll conclude this section with my best piece of fitness advice:

Break a sweat every day doing something you love.

You don't need to, and shouldn't, force yourself to do anything miserable for the sake of your health. Active, unstructured fun is an integral component of a good life. If you don't like anything in particular yet, try a bunch of things. Cross-training, or training for more than one activity at once, is best for balance. My favorites are outside in the fresh air—hiking, trail running, mountain biking, backcountry skiing, swimming, and bouldering. My mom loves daily walks and teaches Zumba at church. My brother Mark stays in great shape tilling dirt as an organic farmer. You might like golf. Cool! Fun is the most important part. Make that happen and your health will take care of itself.

THE SPRINTING ANGELS

For years, I thought I had a useless superpower—I could finish a marathon. But being able to run long distances at a moderate pace doesn't seem to bring much of a competitive advantage in a world swirling with planes, trains, and automobiles. My daily runs were a form of meditation—a bit of "me" time to reconnect with my body and clear my mind. Being able to run quickly was merely a nifty side effect without much tangible benefit.

But while outside for lunch at fellow author and friend Danny Dreyer's ChiRunning workshop on March 29, 2014, I saw a passerby collapse facedown on the sidewalk. His skin was purplish, his tongue was swollen, and he was gasping for air. As another passerby called 911, I sprinted for a quarter mile across the school lot into the school gym to find an emergency responder (incidentally, also a listener to my show) who remarkably had an oxygen tank in the back of his car. We sprinted back to the victim and the EMT administered advanced CPR and used the oxygen tank to keep him breathing. Though weak, the man had a pulse when the ambulance arrived a few minutes later. One of the police officers said that if it weren't for our quick sprinting across the school grounds, the man likely wouldn't have made it.

A few weeks later, I received an e-mail from a TV reporter in Dallas who said a man named Doug had recently survived a heart attack and was searching for the "three angels" who had saved his life. Now recovering from a quadruple bypass, Doug says that he is "living proof that CPR works." Being in great shape isn't just for you, it's part of being a good Samaritan.

PART IV

The Wild Diet

> **Out of clutter, find simplicity.**
>
> —*Albert Einstein*

Famished and thirsty on a sunny afternoon in a small village in Thailand, we happened upon an open-air restaurant. We sat down, saw that *everything* looked good, and ordered an enormous feast, our first meal of the day. A moment later, the cook sprinted out the back of the kitchen with an empty basket. After five minutes, he reappeared with eggs from his neighbor's chickens, veggies from the garden, and spices to make curry from scratch. That's fresh food, and it's the way the healthiest people on earth eat every day.

Once food is picked or packed, it enters a state of rapid decomposition that destroys essential vitamins, minerals, and phytonutrients. When I go back to where I grew up on the old farm in New Hampshire, we make salads and smoothies from the weeds, herbs, spices, fruit, flowers, vegetables, and other plants growing in our backyard. That's what freshness is all about—food that was very Recently Alive and Well (RAW). That means the cow that produced your cheese grazed happily on pasture, your eggs come from chickens eating their natural diet of insects and worms in the backyard, and your seasonal veggies were just picked from an organic garden.

Food is more than the sum of its nutrients. When eaten the right way, according to the laws of nature, food is medicine. Before the Civil War, most families in America were treated by women who collected remedies from nearby woods and streams or grew them in their gardens. One of these women, Martha Ballard, offers a glimpse of what healers like herself believed medicine to be. She writes,

Nature offers solutions to its own problems. Remedies for illness can be found in the earth, in the animal world, and in the human body itself.

Food is the foundation for life. It's meant to nourish and bring your body to its optimal state of health—burning fat, building muscle, and bringing peace of mind. The closer you can get to a food's source—straight from the ground, tree, or carcass—the better.

Is all modern, post-agricultural food harmful, fattening, or unhealthy? Not necessarily, but the Wild Diet follows this principle: Eat plenty of whole and naturally edible foods; and be skeptical of manipulated, processed, and invented food products. This way, your body will burn fat as its main fuel source, returning you to the lean human body that's already a part of your genetic code.

WHAT'S ON THE MENU

Over hundreds of thousands of years, nature has fine-tuned human physiology to thrive on a diet of plants and animals—vegetables, meat, and occasional fruits, nuts, and seeds—which are naturally high in fat, protein, and fiber and relatively low in carbohydrates (also known as carbs). Plants (vegetables, fruits, nuts, seeds, and herbs and spices) and animals (meat, fish, fowl, and eggs) will make up the lion's share of your meals. Nutrient-dense vegetables, fruits, herbs and spices will represent your main source of fibrous carbohydrates and micronutrients (vitamins, minerals, antioxidants, anti-inflammatory agents, and phytonutrients). Raw nuts, seeds, their derivative butters, and animal foods provide nutrient-dense sources of energy, stimulate minimal insulin production, offer the quality forms of healthy protein and fat, and will represent the bulk of your caloric intake.

One of the benefits of Wild foods—especially vegetables, meats, and fruits—is that they are difficult to overeat. Vegetables and fruits provide considerable bulk, fiber, and water, which fill up our stomachs and supply us with energy throughout the day. Protein and fat from meat are also extremely satisfying and keep hunger at bay. Because these foods are digested slowly, they provide steady energy over the day and normalize blood glucose and insulin levels. Aim to eat at least two to three times more plant food by weight as you do eat meat . . . and look forward to feeling very full and satisfied.

One of the best things about eating fresh foods is that they don't take much time, effort, or creativity to taste great. You can eat many vegetables raw—it doesn't get much easier than that. It's hard to screw up fresh, high-quality foods even if you are a hopeless cook.

But please don't take this to mean that you can eat fatty foods *and* lots of quick-burning carbs. If you want to lose fat, you'll want to avoid starches and sugars—pasta, biscuits, toast, hash browns, fries, sweets, and everything else that raises your blood sugar. Don't worry, you still get one "free" meal a week where you can eat whatever you want. And if there is such thing as a "free lunch," it's directly after your workout. After all, cheesecake is good for the soul.

HOW TO BURN FAT WITH WILD FOOD

It's time to return your body to the fat-burning machine it was meant to be. When you burn more energy than you consume, your body releases hormones and enzymes that signal your fat cells to release stored fat (adipose) for energy. The fat cells then empty their contents (called triglycerol) into the bloodstream as free fatty acids. These free fatty acids are then transported through the blood to whatever tissues need energy—including the liver, kidneys, and muscles. Then the glycerol and fatty acids are further broken down within the tissue cells by chemical processes that ultimately produce energy for your body.

Eventually, all that remains from your stored fat deposits is water and carbon dioxide, which your body excretes as urine, sweat, or exhaled air. Pretty cool, right?

If you want to understand fat loss, there's good news and bad news. Which do you want first? Okay. Here's the bad news.

Sugar becomes fat.

And the good news.

Fat becomes energy.

When you follow the Wild Diet, we're going to help your body adapt from a fat-storing "Sugar Burner" to a lean and mean "Fat Burner." How? By avoiding sugar and grains, and eating plenty of delicious veggies, meats, nuts, and legumes instead. I transformed my flabby belly to lean, sculpted abs by eating butter, heavy cream, animal fat, bacon, cheese, nuts, avocado, coconut, and even chocolate. You can, too.

HOW OUR BODIES STORE FAT

From parsnips to pot roast, all food is made up of macronutrients, micronutrients, and water. Macronutrients—proteins, carbohydrates, and fats—provide energy (measured as calories, but only for convenience's sake) to sustain life. While some of each macronutrient is necessary for normal function, each plays a very different role in fat metabolism. Let's get one thing straight: It's not fat that's making most of the developed world store fat—it's carbs. While fats tend to burn clean and provide steady energy for the body, carbs and sugar burn dirty, creating free radicals, accelerating aging, feeding pathogens, and taxing the liver and pancreas in the process.

All carbohydrates break down in your system into glucose (a simple form of sugar), producing a rapid increase in blood sugar. When your blood sugar is elevated from over-consumption of carbs, your pancreas secretes insulin to clear glucose (which is damaging to organs and tissues in excess) from your blood and stores it in liver, muscle, or fat cells.

The body can handle only so many carbs at a time. Once the glycogen storage cells in the liver and muscle are full—as they are nearly all the time in sedentary people since they don't use them as energy for exercise—the remainder of the glucose is converted to and stored as fat.

Your body can either store or burn fat, but not both at the same time. The level of the hormone insulin in your blood dictates whether your body will burn fat (called lipolysis) or store it (called lipogenesis). Specifically, when insulin is elevated, your body is unable to release fat from your fat stores. Keeping carbs low and fasting are the main tools I use to keep insulin levels in check, which allows me to burn stored body fat as well as dietary fat for energy instead of sugar. While fasting and eating low carb enables you to burn fat with ease, chowing on carbs does precisely the opposite.

The primary role of insulin is the storage of nutrients, for better or worse. Insulin also regulates the level of sugar in the blood, induces fat storage, and performs thousands of other tasks within the human body. In excess, insulin can make you hungry, moody, sleepy, bloated, or light-headed. It can also elevate cholesterol, raise blood pressure, cause your body to retain fluid, wreak havoc on your arteries, and convert sugar into fat.

Have you noticed that some people around you tend to gain weight every year even though they haven't changed their diet or exercise habits? In most cases, their weight gain occurs because they are on their way to insulin resistance syndrome (also known as metabolic syndrome or syndrome X), an increasingly common condition that results from long-term overconsumption of carbohydrates and other lifestyle imbalances out of sync with our biology.

Insulin resistance occurs as the body's constant battle to regulate your skyrocketing blood sugar with floods of insulin eventually causes the system to malfunction. (You know that groggy, achy, gross feeling you get just after the sugar high? That's what too much insulin feels like.) Once desensitized, insulin essentially stops working and your body requires *more* of it to properly clear glucose from the bloodstream. As a result, the pancreas pumps out more and more insulin, which creates the constant state of elevated insulin levels in the blood (known as hyperinsulinemia) and low blood sugar (hypoglycemia). This abundance of fat-storing insulin causes people to become fatter and fatter despite eating the same foods they have for years.

This partially explains why some couch-strapped teenagers can drink gallons of soda and eat all the pizza, chips, and donuts they want without gaining weight: Their insulin sensitivity is still intact. As the body ages and insulin resistance eventually kicks in, they suddenly start gaining weight. Some of us can withstand the onslaught of carbs longer than others, but at some point the body just gives up. Eventually, the cells that produce insulin (which are called pancreatic beta cells) burn out.

Once burnt-out pancreatic beta cells are unable to produce sufficient insulin, the body officially has type 2 diabetes, which often leads to nerve damage, blindness, kidney failure, heart attack, and stroke. Type 2 diabetes was once a rare affliction, diagnosed in less than one-tenth of one percent of the population at the turn of the twentieth century. Now, type 2 diabetes is a full-blown epidemic affecting 10 percent of the population and quickly increasing with a price tag of $245 billion a year as of 2012. The good news is this: If you catch it in time, resistance to insulin is reversible.

Insulin isn't all bad. You can even use it to your advantage to shuttle amino acids and glucose to build muscle after an intense workout. In fact, many athletes, bodybuilders, models, and movie stars drop weight by carefully controlling insulin through a cyclical ketogenic diet. You'll see how to use this same strategy to improve body composition on page 311.

Fat

The biggest problem with fat is that it's called "fat." The fact that the fat you eat and the fat that's stored in your body are called by the same name is misleading. The human digestive system is a work of art, and the attempt to explain any whole food in terms of macronutrients often misses the point. While the world of nutrition likes to make things complicated, deciding what to eat for lunch shouldn't be.

You can think of fat as "concentrated energy," providing twice as many calories per gram as protein or carbs. But eating fat isn't *fattening*; in fact, the overwhelming majority of independent studies support a high-fat diet for humans. Compared to those who restrict themselves to a low-fat diet, dieters who eat more fat experience a leaner body composition as well as reduced cholesterol, triglycerides, blood pressure, and other heart disease risk factors. Fat is a fat-burner's best friend.

If food marketers and backward government recommendations have frightened you away from fat, here are some reasons to fall back in love with it. Fat-friendly plans like the Wild Diet increase fat-burning hormones, promote lean muscle growth, inhibit muscle breakdown, and boost production of youth-restoring growth hormone. Short-chain fats, found in coconut oil, promote weight loss and are associated with a decrease in body weight, waist size, and blood triglycerides. Fats protect your body, promote proper cell function, support the release of fat-burning hormones, aid in the absorption of vitamins and minerals, and add flavor to foods. Fats are found in animals, fish, eggs, milk, nuts, and some vegetables and fungi.

During my high-fat experiments on the *Fat-Burning Man* show, I'd drink a cup of heavy cream, fry up eight egg yolks in bacon fat for breakfast, and down full-fat coconut cream by the can. Interestingly, the same biomarkers of health that the fat-phobic might say would go haywire—specifically cholesterol, triglycerides, and C-reactive protein—each came back normal or even improved. I've even been spotted eating grass-fed butter by the stick in a pinch, and I carry around packets of fat as snacks while working or adventuring, which are wonderful for your skin and brain. Fat really isn't as scary as it might seem.

The Truth About Saturated Fat, Cholesterol, and Heart Disease

For decades, Americans have been told that eating saturated fat and cholesterol (found in butter, beef, and other animal fats) clogs arteries and causes heart disease. The justification for the anti–saturated fat propaganda is misguided, however, based upon Ancel Keys's doctored data from the 1950s. In fact, research shows that some saturated fat can actually *decrease* cholesterol, blood pressure, risk of heart disease, and risk of obesity. We've been eating saturated fat safely for thousands of years, as has much of the animal kingdom. It's not fat that's the problem; it's *processed* saturated fat and trans fats that we need to worry about.

Cholesterol, in and of itself, isn't actually bad for you. In fact, almost every cell in the body produces cholesterol. Cholesterol is nature's repair substance and is vital to the function of the brain and nervous system. Many important hormones are made of cholesterol, including the sex hormones testosterone, estrogen, and progesterone, hormones that regulate mineral metabolism and blood sugar, as well as hormones that help us tolerate stress. Cholesterol even acts as a powerful antioxidant that protects us against free radicals and cancer. Suffice it to say that when you eat real food, mostly plants, you don't need to study the science of cholesterol, count calories, or steer clear of eggs to avoid heart disease and achieve great health.

If you're worried about heart disease, know that *eating* cholesterol doesn't necessarily clog your arteries, either. In fact, you're just as likely to have a heart attack with low cholesterol as you are with high cholesterol. And in some studies, high cholesterol is associated with a longer life-span.

Most excess cholesterol is made by the body itself, rather than consumed in the diet. In fact, most Americans consume only about one-third of the amount of cholesterol every day that the body already makes on its own. And much of the cholesterol we consume doesn't even make it into the bloodstream, so if worries about cholesterol have been keeping you away from delicious food, it's time to bring bacon back to breakfast.

The Good Fats We Crave

Our native diet was extremely high in fat—primarily the much-maligned saturated fat. The Inuit enjoyed lives free of heart disease despite sourcing 90 percent or more of their daily calories from fat. Native Americans favored meat from healthy, older animals because they had built up layers of nutrient-dense saturated fat along their backs, which was rendered and stored to provide concentrated energy during the meager seasons.

Our ancestors coveted natural fats and oils like they were liquid gold. Before modern oil processing, our fat was sourced from animals, including butter, lard, tallow, marrow, and from fatty plants like coconut and olive. Unlike polyunsaturated fat, these saturated and monounsaturated fats store well in your pantry and resist oxidization and rancidity.

Our Favorite Fats

Cooking Fats

Cook low and slow and keep the drippings.

- Butter and ghee (particularly from grass-fed cows)
- Animal fats from grass-fed/pastured/wild animals (lard, tallow, duck, etc.)
- Coconut oil
- Avocado oil

Fats to Eat Cold

Since they have a low smoke point and contain delicate omega-3s, eat these fats cold.

- Olive oil
- Fish oils
- Nuts and nut butters
- Flaxseed oil
- Other whole, natural fats

Healthy fat is perfect for curbing the appetite. When I'm hungry or need a boost of energy, I reach for high-fat foods like nuts, eggs, avocado, coconut, and full-fat dairy. At 9 calories per gram, fat is more calorically dense than protein or carbs. That makes it easier to overeat than protein, fruits, or vegetables. Mindlessly pounding sticks of butter, chugging whipping cream, or slurping bacon fat by the spoonful won't do you any favors. Adjust your consumption of fat based on hunger, energy, and exercise levels to find a healthy balance. If your weight begins to drift, you may find that eating more protein or non-starchy vegetables and scaling down your fat intake is more effective for fat loss in your body.

OMEGA-3s

When you eat Wild foods, you'll be getting plenty of brain-boosting, fat-burning omega-3s, a polyunsaturated fat that occurs naturally in oily fish, grass-fed meats and eggs, nuts, seeds, and leafy green vegetables. Omega-3s are anti-inflammatory agents involved in producing energy from food substances and then moving that energy throughout your system. Omega-3s also encourage fat metabolism by regulating insulin levels.

Healthy sources of omega-3s include:

- Wild-caught fish and seafood, especially cold-water fish such as salmon, mackerel, halibut, and herring
- Pasture-raised poultry and their eggs
- Pasture-raised ruminant animals, such as cows, bison, and lamb
- Pasture-raised liver and organ meats
- Flax- and chia seeds and their oil, which can be used as an ingredient in salad dressings, poured over vegetables, or used as a supplement
- Walnuts and macadamia nuts
- Leafy green vegetables

Fats to Avoid

Avoid anything that is processed, packaged, or fried—especially processed foods containing newfangled trans fats, hydrogenated fats, and polyunsaturated oils. This includes shortening, margarine, and industrial seed oils (e.g., corn, cottonseed, soybean, safflower, and canola). It's not just processed vegetable fats that cause problems, though. Industrial animal fats are best avoided, as well.

While fat from healthy animals is nutrient dense and beneficial for your health, fat from sick animals isn't. Since cows, poultry, and fish are fed high-carb, GMO, non-native diets in industrial feedlots and fish farms, its best to avoid fat from conventional meat. Like humans, animals store antibiotics, feed pesticides, synthetic growth hormones, and other toxins in their fat stores. If you're eating conventional meat that may come from a sick animal, trim or drain off any excess fat to avoid toxins.

PROTEIN

Protein will be one of your best weapons to reach and maintain your ideal body composition. If you want to curb hunger and lose weight rapidly without feeling deprived, eat more high-quality protein—up to 1 gram per pound of your ideal body weight daily. Consuming plenty of protein does more than just keep you feeling full, it actually helps build your muscles, organs, and brain. As the only food constituent containing nitrogen, protein forms the basic building blocks of human matter and is essential to growth and repair of the body.

Eating protein propels anabolism (muscle-building), decreases risk of catabolism (muscle-wasting), and actually increases your resting metabolic rate by producing body heat (known as thermogenesis). Protein also boosts your overall health by improving immunity and antioxidant function and enhancing insulin function. Protein is found in many foods, notably meats, fish, seafood, eggs, and dairy, as well as vegetables, beans, nuts, legumes, and fungi.

You can eat as much protein as you'd like, but make it high quality. Don't be afraid of eating too much protein as long as it's in the form of whole food. Go for grass-finished, pastured, wild, local game, and organic meats over conventionally raised and processed meats. In a pinch, unsweetened protein shakes or bars can help get the protein you need, but it's always best to go with real food.

During digestion, your body breaks food down into energy. In order to access this energy, the body must *expend* energy. Protein requires two and a half to three times more energy to digest than carbohydrates or fat. This means that the same caloric intake of protein burns more energy than an equal amount of fat or carbs, resulting in rapid fat loss. This is known as thermogenesis, and it's one of the reasons you'd need to eat twice as much protein to get the equivalent caloric energy in the same amount of fat.

Is it possible to eat too much protein? Theoretically, yes. The protein ceiling falls somewhere around 40 percent of your caloric intake. However, since protein is very filling and only contains 4 calories per gram (as opposed to 9 calories per gram in fat or 7 calories per gram in alcohol), unless you're drinking a lot of protein shakes, eating protein bars, or overdoing supplements, that 40 percent of your protein intake is nearly impossible to overreach.

If you are physically active or trying to build muscle, eat at least 50 to 100 grams of protein a day and up to 1 gram of protein per pound of ideal body weight. This amount of protein will help you increase your lean muscle, especially if you are engaging in high-intensity training as recommended.

The protein in a palm-size portion of meat adds up quickly:

- 6 ounces of lean beef or turkey has upward of 50 grams of protein
- 6 ounces of tuna has 40 grams of protein
- 1 cup of cottage cheese has 28 grams of protein
- 1 cup of lentils has 9 grams of protein
- 1 egg has 6 grams of protein

When you prepare a meal, build it around pastured, grass-fed, or wild-caught animal protein and fibrous vegetables and boost your energy intake and add flavor with nutrient-dense fat. Try to get at least a few bites of a protein-rich food in each meal. It may go against your habits and conditioning, but I cannot overemphasize the importance of eating plenty of protein for fat loss; building strong, toned muscle; and a lean body composition. Fear steak no longer.

CARBOHYDRATES

Most people overeat carbs, especially the bad kind. Anthropologists estimate that many of our hunter-gathering ancestors consumed fewer than 100 grams of net carbs a day, primarily from fruits and vegetables. In stark contrast, the typical American consumes *350 to 600 grams a day* primarily from various sugar and grain products. As carbohydrates are primarily responsible for enabling fat storage, it is not difficult to see why many of us are overweight.

Imagine filling two cups with pure, white sugar and spooning it into your mouth one bite at a time. Believe it or not, that's the amount of simple sugar your body metabolizes every day if you source 60 percent of your calories from carbs, as most of us do. Bread, pasta, cereal, potatoes, rice, fruit, dessert, candy, and so many more: They are all carbohydrates that your body converts to a simple form of sugar called glucose to be readily stored in muscle or as fat.

As far as your body is concerned, processed carbs *are* sugar. Since sugar rots your teeth, accelerates aging, and feeds cancer cells, it's best not to have too much of it. If there is anything worth counting, it's carbs. Limiting carb intake maximizes fat burning and helps to regulate blood sugar and insulin levels. But all carbs are not created equal.

There are three main categories of carbs:

Sugar: Found in concentrates, powders, syrups, and fruit

Starch: Found in roots, tubers, cereals, and grains.

Fiber: Found in roughage, vegetables, fruits, nuts, seeds, and whole grains. Roughage is essential to keeping your digestive tract in good working order.

The total number of carbohydrates listed on nutrition labels is not the whole story. It's *net* carbs that really matter, since total carbs includes fiber. Fiber from fruit and veggies is beneficial—fiber feeds your probiotic gut bacteria, detoxifies your digestive tract, and gives you steady energy throughout the day.

Count your *net* carbs, not your total carbs. To calculate net carbs, simply subtract the dietary fiber content from the total carbs.

Carbs – Fiber = Net Carbs

Limiting net carbs to 50 to 100 grams per day accelerates fat burning for most people. For what it's worth, for bodybuilding, Arnold Schwarzenegger recommended consuming just 60 to 100 grams of net carbs a day, with the rest of calories coming from fat and protein. Hard to argue with the Terminator.

As long as you limit starches, sugars, and fruit, it's difficult to exceed 100 grams of net carbs in a day even if you eat generous amounts of colorful vegetables and a few servings of fruit.

"HAVE YOU CONSUMED RICE TODAY?"

On a visit to the small Indonesian island of Bali, our guide brought us to paddies and plantations to sample numerous strains of ancient rice. Our favorite, red rice, is a long grain with a deep reddish-brown hue on the outside and a white center. When you cook it just right (low and slow), this chewy and wholesome rice adopts the fluffy texture of old-fashioned whole-grain oats.

Like other grains, many modern strains of rice have been domesticated and bred for characteristics that have little to do with your health. Low-quality rice even contains "troubling" levels of arsenic, a known carcinogen and poison. However, many healthful ancient strains of rice are readily available at health food stores, Asian markets, in some supermarkets, and online.

Wild rice (actually an edible grass) is relatively easy to find and tastes more nutty and substantial than the overcooked mush that comes out of an ice cream scoop at many restaurants in America. Unlike processed white rice, whole-grain rice—like brown, black, and red—leaves the bran intact, making for a more nutritious grain. Both brown and red rice can be long-, medium- or short-grain. Long-grain rice is drier and fluffs when cooked. Short-grain rice has higher starch content and is sticky when cooked.

In most of the world, rice isn't just a side dish, it's a part of life. In the Thai language, "How are you?" translates roughly to "Have you consumed rice today?"

As we whizzed through the magnificent rolling rice paddies while touring through Bali, our guide and driver explained: "Almost all of our rice is still grown by hand, not machines. Many farmers here." More than food, rice is considered sacred and often plays a fundamental role in Balinese offerings and ceremonies.

"How do Americans grow rice?" our driver inquired, glancing in the rearview mirror as we narrowly escaped a head-on collision with a speeding truck hauling hand-woven baskets.

"With big machines, cheap oil, and lots of pesticides," I admitted. "But we're working on that."

How Many Carbs Should I Eat?

For most people, the best range for healthy fat loss is 50 to 100 grams of net carbs a day, perhaps more if you're especially physically active. But you don't need to "count carbs" because it's easy to stay well within 50 to 150 grams on the Wild Diet—even when you eat loads of colorful vegetables and a fair amount of fruit. It's difficult to stay in this range, however, when you consume modern foods such as grains, processed foods, or sugars.

In modest amounts, carbs are not your enemy. Consuming carbs from fruits and vegetables is necessary to achieve optimal body function and balance—especially if you are physically active, have a high metabolism, or have a low tolerance for fat or protein. Moderate consumption of slow-burning carbs and starches promotes healthy body function by providing your brain with glucose (brain fuel) and your liver and muscles with glycogen (muscle fuel) and helps regulate circadian rhythms to help you sleep, especially when you eat carbs at night.

The more active you are, the better your body can utilize and dispose of carbs. So if you have a very active metabolism or you are an athlete, don't be afraid of fueling up with slow-burning starches and carbs like boiled sweet potatoes, whole-grain rice, quinoa, and other whole Wild foods. But be careful—eating carbs in excess of your glycogen stores will risk fat storage, despite large amounts of exercise. This is easy to do when you come back from your long runs and eat a whole pie. Been there, done that.

SLOW-BURNING VS. QUICK-BURNING CARBS

The Glycemic Index (GI) is a rating system that evaluates how different foods affect blood sugar levels—essentially, it's a rough indicator of the likelihood that eating that food will make you store fat, with lower numbers being more favorable for fat burning. High-GI carbohydrates, such as white bread, sugar, cereal, and most other processed food, burn quickly, spike your blood sugar, and cause a flood of insulin that triggers your body to store fat and become hungry again within an hour or two.

In contrast, slow-burning starches and lower-GI foods, such as vegetables, cut your appetite and keep you satisfied for hours on end. These slow-burning carbs are more efficient at keeping glucose levels stabilized and insulin in check. The Wild Diet prioritizes slow-burning carbohydrates with low GIs to ensure more consistent and long-lasting energy and reduced fat storage.

When to Eat Carbs

The best time to eat carbs is in the evening, as carbs cue your body to enter "rest and digest" mode and help you fall asleep. Most people lose the most fat when avoiding carbs in the morning in favor of a high-fat or high-protein breakfast instead. Think "gatherer" by day—light snacking on low-glycemic veggies, nuts, and fruit—and "hunter" by night, with a hearty source of protein, plenty of fat, and slow-burning carbs like whole-grain rice or sweet potato. For example, I might snack on raw carbs like veggies and fruit during the day, but tend to avoid cooked carbs until late afternoon or evening.

Consuming carbs within sixty to ninety minutes immediately following intervals, strength training, or other intense physical activity will aid recovery and refuel glycogen stores for your next session. After an intense workout, your body is primed to absorb nutrients, and insulin helps shunt extra carb calories to help replenish and grow muscle tissue. I often work out fasted and eat a carb- and protein-heavy meal directly after. See the "Fasting and Feasting" section on pages 55 to 69 for more details.

VITAMINS

Vitamins have an essential role not only in maintaining the health of the body but in protection from illness and disease. Science has discovered more than 40 different vitamins, of which about a dozen are essential for humans. Vitamin D can be synthesized by the skin when exposed to sunlight, and gut bacteria can synthesize vitamin K, but many vitamins must be obtained from food.

A well-nourished person generally carries a month's supply of vitamins in their body. Of those, vitamin C is the first that needs to be replenished (lest you get a mean case of scurvy like a sea-weary pirate, or my roommate in college who subsisted almost exclusively on ramen noodles). The second vitamin to replenish is vitamin A, which aids vision and prevents eye disease. Eat a wide variety of herbs and spices, and fresh seasonal fruits and vegetables to ensure you get the full spectrum of nutrients you need to thrive.

MINERALS AND TRACE ELEMENTS

Minerals have vital roles in body functions. We require a steady quantity of certain minerals to function normally, including magnesium, calcium, sulphur, phosphorus, sodium, and potassium. Other minerals are required in smaller amounts, including iodine, iron, and flourine.

Unfortunately, decades of unsustainable farming practices have caused the amount of minerals in our soil—and our food—to plummet. We counter this lack of minerals in our soil by consuming bone broth weekly and supplementing with bulkier minerals such as magnesium in powdered form. To improve taste and nutrition, add a few drops of trace minerals to your drinking water.

VARIETY, THE SPICE OF LIFE

Many fat-loss programs recommend that you eat the same meals every month, every week, or even every day, often because they want to sell you their microwave dinners, protein bars, and shakes. Gym rats might argue that it's "easier to hit your macros" when you eat the same thing every day. But that's terrible advice, and here's why.

Not only will eating the same thing every day bore you to tears, but you'll also be missing out on the wide spectrum of nutrients naturally found in seasonal foods. When you let what naturally grows during the season dictate what you put on your plate—tomatoes in the summer and apples in September, for example—your fresh produce will be more satisfying and filling because the harvest contains the cycle of nutrients your body needs to thrive. The more you incorporate variety into your nutritional habits, the healthier and happier you'll be.

While hunter-gatherers in the Australian outback today live on eight hundred varieties of wild plant foods, Americans live principally on three industrial crops: corn, soy, and wheat. Since we're missing out on the majority of foods that our ancestors once ate, many of us are deficient in critical vitamins and minerals, including vitamin D, vitamin K, magnesium, and zinc, to name a few.

What gave hunter-gatherers perfect teeth, lean frames, and disease-free bodies? They relished nutrient-dense delicacies like beaver tail, stewed bonemeal pudding, and fermented caribou intestines stuffed with organ meats. You don't have much use for multivitamins when you eat food like that.

Fortunately, fermented caribou intestine isn't the only nutrient-dense food out there.

One of the easiest ways to get more variety in your diet is by looking at your traditional family recipes. What did your grandparents eat? Were there strange soups, cod livers, or fermented vegetables fizzing in the cupboard? Perhaps you'll find old family recipes for nutrient-dense meals like liver and onions, sausage, or haggis. Get in touch with your relatives and dust off that family cookbook to see what you can bring back to life.

The body's ability to absorb nutrients is dictated by the presence or absence of cofactors, critical substances that "unlock" the nutrition in food to be utilized by the body, and many traditional food preparations and dishes are designed to keep our bodies healthy. For example, eating cheese with eggs can increase uptake of vitamin D; eating wasabi and ginger with raw fish protects against bacteria, viruses, and disease; and soaking and sprouting nuts, seeds, and grains, as our ancestors once did, reduces antinutrients like lectins and phytates that can damage the gut and releases enzymes that help our bodies gain access to their nutrients.

Nutrients from real food are vastly superior to synthetic and added vitamins and minerals—it's difficult, expensive, and some would argue impossible to compensate for a poor diet through supplementation. As such, it's essential to aim for fresh, high-quality foods that are naturally high in micronutrients to achieve optimal health.

THE CURIOUS CASE OF POTTENGER'S CATS

Dr. Francis Pottenger Jr. was a veterinarian who worked in a lab that produced adrenal hormones and tested them on cats. The death rate of Pottenger's cats was high, but he noticed when the offal portion of their diet—liver, tripe, sweetbreads, brains, and heart—was served raw rather than cooked, the health of the cats improved markedly.

Beginning in 1932, Pottenger conducted a remarkable ten-year experiment that evaluated five diets over four generations, including nine hundred cats. He found that cats fed raw milk, raw meat, and offal maintained health throughout four generations of breeding. However, the cats that ate only cooked meat and pasteurized, evaporated, or condensed milk experienced steadily deteriorating health.

- First-generation cats developed degenerative diseases late in life.
- Second-generation cats developed degenerative diseases in midlife.
- Third-generation cats developed diseases, allergies, and soft bones and succumbed to parasitic infections early in life. Most of the cats could not produce offspring.
- Not a single fourth-generation cat could reproduce. Fourth-generation cats suffered almost all of the medically documented human degenerative diseases.

It's now generally accepted that the decline in health of Pottenger's cats was due to nutritional deficiencies induced by cooking and processing, which destroys taurine, an essential nutrient for cats. High-temperature processing techniques like pasteurization and homogenization destroy nutrients in a similar manner. For tips on how to feed your pets their native diet, see page 316.

GO FRESH, LOCAL, ORGANIC, AND IN-SEASON

Go organic when you can—remember, all food was once organic. Today, certified organic crops have a higher standard of quality and are required to be grown in safe soil, have no modifications, and must remain separate from conventional products. Organic farmers are not allowed to use synthetic pesticides, bioengineered genes (GMOs), petroleum-based fertilizers, or sewage sludge–based fertilizers. Organic foods have fewer pesticides, synthetic fertilizers, growth hormones, and antibiotics, and contain higher levels of nutrients than conventional foods. Conventional growers make no such promises.

As such, it is important to go for fresh, organic plants and animals when you can. Honor the natural cycles of the seasons and save a few bucks by purchasing foods that are local and fresh, like cucumbers in the summer, apples in September, and corn in late spring.

Why Heirloom Produce and Heritage Livestock Are Better Than Conventional

Have you ever sliced into a deep pink tomato with white stripes? Perhaps you've eaten carrots that are nearly blue, or a small spiky, bulbous cucumber with a long, spindly vine? If so, you probably know that heirloom varieties of fruits and vegetables are not only beautiful, they're delicious. By definition, heirloom varieties come from seeds that have been passed down from generation to generation and have been allowed to reproduce naturally (think "the opposite of dwarf wheat and GMOs"). Generally speaking, these varieties of fruits and vegetables are more nutritionally dense (you can tell by their deep and varied coloration) than their conventional counterparts. Plus, they are usually locally grown and have been allowed to ripen on the vine, making them more tasty and nutritious.

Heirloom livestock are also quite different from the cows, pigs, and chickens you find on a factory farm. Heirloom chickens are beautiful—speckled red and brown, sleek black with dapples of gray, or maybe a deep chocolate brown—and they come in countless colors and look nothing like the pure white, extra-large-breasted chickens packed into factory-farm cages. These poor conventional animals, such as the enormous turkeys many of us eat during the holidays, are bred to have breasts so large that their feet would break if they attempted to walk during adulthood.

Heritage livestock, however, from chickens and pigs to cows and sheep, are more capable of withstanding the elements and have a stronger immune system, making it so they do not need antibiotics to survive and thrive like their conventional cousins. Heritage livestock is often raised organic and fed their natural diet, making their eggs, dairy, and meat more nutritious than conventional. Remember: The healthier the animal you eat, the healthier you'll be.

After trying some truly strange exotic fruits and vegetables in distant lands, I've learned this: The weirder it looks, the better it tastes. Get your tomatoes ugly.

EAT LIKE THE LOCALS

While sampling raw cacao, fresh heirloom chile pepper, local tobacco, and cat poop coffee at a plantation on the Indonesian island of Bali, I chatted with two locals about how they eat at home. Despite the fact that nearly every restaurant, villa, and resort brings visitors a whopping glass of tropical fruit juice, the locals don't bother.

"We're too lazy to make juice!" our friend Nyoman says. "Fruit turns to juice in stomach anyway. We just eat fruit," he says, smiling. "We sometimes take two meals a day, with no breakfast. But usually we eat fried banana with Bali coffee in the morning."

"How about lunch and dinner?"

"We cook vegetables, rice, and maybe meat or fish. We only need a few bites. Not like the Americans who eat half a chicken. . . . A little chicken leg feeds our whole family!" Nyoman exclaims as our guide, Wayan, nods in approval.

As any local will tell you, the heavy, rich meals offered at the restaurants are meals that you wouldn't find at home in daily practice. They cook one meal a day—vegetables, rice, and meat—and eat it around noon. In the evening, they don't use microwaves. Like the fresh eggs at their village markets, they eat their food at room temperature with the rest of their family. We found that cooking meals in advance and eating food at room temperature saves time and takes the stress out of family dinners.

"What advice would you give someone who gets fat here to lose weight?" I ask, now crying from the chiles.

"Always give them fresh food," Nyoman explains. "Anyone who eats too much food from boxes gets fat."

GREENS: THE ONE THING EVERY HEALTH EXPERT AGREES ABOUT

Although health experts squabble about everything else, there is one thing about which almost every health expert worth his or her salt agrees—that we should all eat more fresh green vegetables. Above all else, healthy people make it a priority to get their greens every day, and you should, too.

I eat an enormous amount of vegetables, as often as I can—usually several times a day, which takes deliberate effort. Raw veggie addiction is much like beer, coffee, and smoking: I crave greens every day and get cranky without them. That's where you want to be. Push through the first few days of salad eating until you're hooked.

HOW TO MAKE A GREEN SMOOTHIE

It's a versatile, delicious, nutritional powerhouse that is incredibly easy to make. The most effective fat-burning breakfast on the face of the Earth is the green smoothie.

The nutritional equivalent of eating a salad and then some, green smoothies are packed with vitamins and minerals, water, satiating fiber, and raw food enzymes to aid digestion. Green smoothies are detoxifying and alkalizing, which restores balance within your body to burn off fat and restore health.

Store-bought "green smoothies" from the bottle are almost always devoid of fiber and packed with preservatives and sugar. Avoid them and make your own—it will taste better, be better for you, and save you money.

Combine the following four categories of ingredients to taste:

- Green vegetable (use one or more): kale, spinach, bok choy, collard greens, cabbage greens, Swiss chard, beet greens, sprouts, cucumber, broccoli, celery, avocado
- Liquid (use one): water, tea, almond milk, coconut milk, coconut water, raw milk, kefir. Add ice if you like your smoothie chilled.
- Fruit (limit to one serving of low-sugar fruit like berries if fat loss is the goal, fresh or frozen): strawberries, blueberries, bananas, apples, cherries, coconut, carrots, beets (top and root), lemon, ginger root, pumpkin, tomatoes
- Add-ins: protein powder (with no added sugar), flax meal (for omega-3s), cinnamon (regulates blood sugar), stevia, spirulina, chlorella, hulled hemp seeds, chia seeds soaked in water, olive oil, powdered vitamin C

Do you *need* to drink green smoothies? Absolutely not. Really, if we would just *eat* our daily salads, we wouldn't have to blend them up in some ridiculous contraption. But green smoothies are great if you're in a hurry or if you don't find yourself eating a daily salad. If you'd rather drink your salad than eat it, give it a whirl.

MEAT, FOWL, AND EGGS

While drifting down a river in Fiji where *Anacondas* (the movie about enormous man-eating snakes) was filmed, Alyson and I spotted a giant beast scrambling down the cliffs. Muscular and graceful, this magnificent animal bounded to the riverbank and burst through the jungle below. It was . . . a cow.

"I've never seen a cow like that," I said to my Fijian guide. "It's like a supercow."

He chuckled. "Yes, wild cow. We let them loose in the jungle when they're babies and they live in the jungle. When they're big enough, we call them back and have a feast. Our cows have good lives here."

Meet Your Meat

If you believe that the animals your chicken nuggets are made from have ever seen the light of day or felt grass under their feet, you are living a fantasy of bygone times. Today, factory-farmed animals are not treated humanely, but Big Food does its best to keep that a secret. As shoppers, we're encouraged to distance ourselves from the animals we're eating as much as possible. But if you take the time to befriend a backyard cow, you'll look at your burger differently.

When you eat beef, you're not just eating the cow, you're consuming the entire food chain. If the cow that became your burger lived on food it's not meant to eat, like the corn fed to conventional cattle to fatten them quickly, and survived on a steady dose of antibiotics and growth hormones, you're eating the meat of a sick animal. The toxic, marbled meat from blubbery feedlot cows, for example, bears little resemblance to meat from the powerful aurochs (wild cows) and buffalo our ancestors ate in the natural world.

Meat from wild animals typically carry little external fat, nearly no fat between the muscles, and contain very few toxins. In stark contrast, feedlot animals are fat and sick, with several inches of white fat covering their bodies. Despite the fact that the FDA has known about the health risks for nearly fifty years, it's common for factory farms to feed their cows industrial poultry litter (yes, bird poop) as a staple of their diet. When you eat conventional meat, these toxins, chemicals, and hormones in the meat transfer their negative effects to you.

Production lines often move too quickly for the limited staff in conventional slaughterhouses. Hiccups and minor mishaps in the rapid assembly-line disembowelment of conventionally raised cattle often leads to feces in the meat. This is the root cause of food poisoning from E. coli contamination, which is a daily occurrence across America and one of the principal reasons our meat is banned in other countries. In addition, while the fat from wild or pasture-raised animals is healthy and high in brain-boosting omega-3 fatty acids, the fat of conventionally raised animals is toxic.

Always buy the cleanest and highest-quality meat (free of hormones, additives, preservatives, artificial coloring agents, etc.) you can find and afford. Game meats and pasture-raised organic animals raised in their natural environment are best. If you eat factory-farmed meat, know that the fat is where the majority of the animal's toxins are stored. Go for a lean cut and trim off the fat before cooking.

One of our favorite things about eating Wild: We save money on grass-finished meat by eating the whole animal, nose to tail, as our ancestors once did. The cuts with the highest nutrient density are actually the organs, not the muscle meat. In fact, many hunter-gatherers, after claiming their kill, ate the prized organs like the liver raw in the field to replenish their energy, accessing its vast spectrum of nutrients after a long hunt. If there was too much to carry, hunters often left the muscle meat, the least nutrient-dense part of the animal, behind in favor of fatty cuts and organ meats.

In the animal kingdom, this is referred to as the "high-grading" of food. During salmon runs in Alaska, grizzly bears do the same, eating only the livers and leaving the rest of the fish on the riverbank. According to the National Park Service,

> If you see bears only eating the skin, brains, and eggs of a salmon, they are practicing good energy economics. At these times, a bear's profit margin in calories is so high that it can ignore some excess fish. As a bear fills up on salmon, it can "afford" to not eat certain parts of the fish. This behavior has been nicknamed "high-grading." Like miners looking for high-grade ore, bears try to consume high-grade fat.
>
> Salmon are a high-calorie meal for a bear. A sockeye salmon contains about 4,500 calories, but the fattiest parts of the fish contain the most calories proportionally. Bears know this and prefer to eat the skin, brain, and eggs—the fattiest parts of a salmon—when fish are in abundance.

If you're looking to save a buck at the farmers' market, this is great news for you. While you might get sticker shock from premium cuts of grass-fed meat, many farmers are willing to part with their fatty offcuts and organ meat for less than half of the price of their steaks. When you learn how to prepare offcuts, like stew meat, meaty bones, and organs, supply and demand often works in your favor. To get the most bang for your buck, ask for marrow bones (for soup and for the dog when she's good), roasts, liver, heart, chicken feet, fish stock bones, and offcuts that you can throw in chili or a stew.

Eggs

Whole eggs from healthy fowl are among the most nutritious foods on earth. Within the walls of its shell, an egg contains enough nutrients to transform a single fertilized cell into a chirping chick in twenty-one days.

In spite of that, the fat-free fad misled nutritionists and doctors into telling us to give up eggs since they contain cholesterol and saturated fat. But as we learned on page 97, cholesterol in food is not at all the same thing as the cholesterol that clogs arteries. One Harvard study found that healthy men and women could eat seven eggs a day with no increased risk of heart disease. That's a lot of quiche.

Eggs are an excellent source of high-quality fat and protein, making them an economical and healthful staple. Scrambled, poached, hard-boiled, Benedict, or baked into homemade desserts, we usually eat several eggs a day in one form or another. If you're bored with chicken eggs, branch out and experiment with quail eggs (tiny and tasty) or duck eggs (big and buttery).

For best nutrition, choose eggs from free-roaming poultry in pasture on their natural diet of insects, seeds, and fruits. The better the diet of your chicken, the more nutrients in your eggs. Pastured eggs are particularly high in choline, an essential nutrient critical to brain function that 90 percent of Americans don't get enough of. Egg yolks are also the richest sources of lutein and zeaxanthin, antioxidants that keep eyes healthy and protect them from the leading cause of blindness, macular degeneration. Eggs are loaded with other vital nutrients, including folate, riboflavin, selenium, and B vitamins.

How to Choose Your Eggs

Buying eggs is confusing, isn't it? Which is better: organic, pasture-raised, or omega-3 enriched? Are farm-fresh eggs really more healthful than conventional? While each